NNSDO national nurs staff development organization

AMERICAN NURSES ASSOCIATION

D0485666

NURSING PROFESSIONAL DEVELOPMENT: SCOPE AND STANDARDS OF PRACTICE

NATIONAL NURSING STAFF DEVELOPMENT ORGANIZATION

AMERICAN NURSES ASSOCIATION
SILVER SPRING, MARYLAND
2010

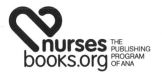

nurses THE PUBLISHING PROGRAM OF ANA
books.org

Library of Congress Cataloging-in-Publication data

National Nursing Staff Development Organization.
Nursing professional development: scope and standards of practice / National Nursing
    Staff Development Organization, American Nurses Association.
        p. ; cm.
Rev. ed. of: Nursing professional development: scope and standards of practice.
    American Nurses Association. ©2000.
    Includes bibliographical references and index.
    ISBN-13: 978-1-55810-272-9 (softcover)
    ISBN-10: 1-55810-272-8 (softcover)
        1. Nursing—Study and teaching (Continuing education)—Standards—United States.
    2. Nurses—In-service training—Standards—United States.   3 [DNLM: 1. Education,
    Nursing, Continuing—standards—United States.   2. Nursing—standards—United
    States.   3. Staff Development—standards—United States.   WY 18.5 S422 2010]

RT76.S366 2010
610.73'071'55—dc21   2010-042007

The American Nurses Association (ANA) is a national professional association. This ANA publication—*Nursing Professional Development: Scope and Standards of Practice*—reflects the thinking of the nursing profession on various issues and should be reviewed in conjunction with state board of nursing policies and practices. State law, rules, and regulations govern the practice of nursing, while *Nursing Professional Development: Scope and Standards of Practice* guides nurses in the application of their professional skills and responsibilities.

Published by Nursesbooks.org
The Publishing Program of ANA
http://www.Nursesbooks.org/

American Nurses Association
8515 Georgia Avenue, Suite 400
Silver Spring, MD 20910-3492
1-800-274-4ANA
http://www.Nursingworld.org/

Design: Scott Bell, Arlington, VA ~ Freedom by Design, Alexandria, VA ~ Stacy Maguire, Sterling, VA … Editorial services: Grammarians, Inc, Washington, DC: Francis Taylor (copyediting) ~ Kelly Saxton (proofreading) ~ Gina Wiatrowski (indexing) … Typesetting: House of Equations, Inc., Arden, NC… Printing: Harris Lithographics, Landover, MD.

First printing July 2010. Second printing February 2011.

ISBN-13: 978-1-55810-272-9   SAN: 851-3481   6M   02/2011R

CONTRIBUTORS

Work Group Members

Dora Bradley, PhD, RN-BC (Chair)

M. Beth Benedict, DrPH, JD, RN

Sandra K. Cesario, PhD, RN-C, FAAN

Mary Harper, PhD, RN-BC

Sheree Henson, MSN, RN, LCCE

Deborah Lindell, DNP, APRN-BC, CNE

Patricia R. Messmer, PhD, RN-BC, FAAN

Judy Morgan, MSN, RN

Gwen Thoma, EdD, RN, NE-BC

Karen Tomajan, MS, RN, NEA-BC

Janice A. Ward, MSN, RN

Chris Wilson, MSN, RN-BC

Debra M. Wolf, PhD, RN

Vanessa Worsham, MSN, APRN, ACNS-BC

NNSDO Staff

Patricia Barlow, BA and Elizabeth Bennett Bailey, BFA, Executive Directors

ANA Staff

Carol Bickford, PhD, RN-BC – Content editor

Katherine Brewer, MSN, RN – Content editor

Maureen Cones, Esq. – Legal counsel

Yvonne Humes, MSA – Project coordinator

Eric Wurzbacher – Project editor

About the Work Group

M. Beth Benedict, DrPH, JD, RN
Social Science Research Analyst, Office of Research, Development and Information, Centers for Medicare and Medicaid Services

Dr. Benedict brought to this workgroup 15 years of experience in continuing education for public health nursing in the American Public Health Association/Public Health Nursing Section. Her research projects include Medicaid-covered women and their children, with a focus on asthma prevention and management. She currently serves as the APHA/PHN lead nurse for its ANCC-accredited provider and approver CE programs.

Dora Bradley PhD, RN-BC
Vice President, Nursing Professional Development, Baylor Health Care System, Dallas TX

In over 25 years of experience in staff development, continuing education, and academic education, Dr. Bradley has worked extensively in measurement in terms of competency, program evaluation, and educational outcomes. She is active in several professional organizations and has served on the NNSDO board of directors. Dr. Bradley also consults on professional practice models and the strategies for integrating such models and bedside evidence-based practices.

Sandra K. Cesario, PhD, MS, RN-C, FAAN
Professor, PhD Program Coordinator, Texas Woman's University–Houston, College of Nursing

Dr. Cesario is a specialist in women's and newborn health with over 30 years of national and international clinical, research, education, and policy development experience. Instrumental in developing and teaching the Nurse Residency Program for the USPHS Indian Health Service, she currently is a consultant to the Association of Women's Health, Obstetric, and Neonatal Nurses (AWHONN) in creating and revising their standards documents, and evidence-based clinical practice guidelines.

Mary G. Harper, PhD, RN-BC
Academic Mentor and Clinical Faculty, Western Governors University, Salt Lake City, UT

With over 30 years experience in nursing and certified in nursing professional development, Dr. Harper's NPD positions have included unit-based educator, education director for a three-hospital system, and mentor for clinical faculty in a university setting. Formally recognized at the national and state levels, a contributor to the Core Curriculum for Staff Development, Dr. Harper's current research is on emotional intelligence in staff nurses and nursing students.

Sheree Henson, MSN RN LCCE
Clinical Education Specialist at Texas Health Harris Methodist Hospital Southwest Fort Worth (THSW)

With over 15 years as a clinical and community educator, Ms. Henson is responsible for the continuous learning services labor and delivery, postpartum, newborn nursery, NICU, med-surg and med-surg telehealth. Recognized by the Dallas-Fort Worth Hospital Councils and the Texas Nurses Association, her current projects include preparing parents for childbirth and implementing the Baby Friendly Hospital Initiative.

Deborah F. Lindell, DNP, RN, PHCNS-BC, CNE
Assistant Professor; Director, Graduate Entry Program; Frances Payne Bolton School of Nursing, Case Western Reserve University

Dr. Lindell's 20+ years of experience as a nurse educator includes 7 years as administrator of a graduate entry nursing program. Certified as an academic nurse educator and clinical nurse specialist in public health nursing, she teaches at the pre-licensure, advanced, and practice doctorate levels. Active in the National League for Nursing's Academic Nurse Educator Certification Program and a consultant to the program, she was also the lead author of NLN's *Scope of Practice for Academic Nurse Educators.*

Patricia R. Messmer, PhD, RN-BC, FAAN
Director of Patient Care Services Research, Children's Mercy Hospitals and Clinics, Kansas City, MO

Dr. Messmer taught in several nursing schools before taking her first directorship (in nursing research and education) in 1989. She continues to work in professional development and other staff development and continuing education activities. Certified in ANCC Nursing Professional Development and has been an ANCC Magnet Appraiser® since 2001, Dr. Messmer serves in leadership roles in several organizations. She received the 2010 Jessie M. Scott Award of the American Nurses Foundation for her career focus on the interdependence among nursing education, practice, and research.

Judith Morgan, MSN, RN
Staff Development Specialist, Good Samaritan Hospital, Vincennes, IN

In her current position at a Magnet® designated facility, Ms. Morgan has dedicated her career to improving patient care and nursing practice. A long-active member of the Indiana State Nurses Association (ISNA), she serves both as her facility's liaison to the continuing education and as chair of its continuing education committee. For the past 10 years she has functioned as AHA Training Center Coordinator, Regional Faculty.

Gwen Beaudean Thoma, EdD, RN, NE-BC
Director of Educational Services, Southeast Missouri Hospital, Cape Girardeau, MO

An education director at Southeast since 1982, Dr. Thoma has over 36 years of leadership experience and is ANCC-certified as a Nurse Executive. She established and still directs the patient education programs for the hospital, and has published and presented nationally. Widely recognized for her career contributions, Dr. Thoma serves on her facility's Magnet Steering Committee, having contributed to its Magnet designation.

Karen Tomajan, MS, RN, NEA-BC
Clinical and Regulatory Consultant, INTEGRIS Baptist Medical Center, Oklahoma City, OK

Throughout her career, Ms. Tomajan has been active in quality, nursing education, and staff development. Past-president of the Oklahoma Nurses Association, she is also active in a number of professional organizations and currently serves on the OJIN Editorial Advisory Board. She is a frequent presenter at conferences on quality, nursing practice and professional development.

Janice A. Ward, MSN, RN
Director of Lifelong Learning, Indiana University School of Nursing

A nurse educator with more than 35 years of experience as a director and clinical instructor in staff development, faculty, and director of education, Ms. Ward's work has included traditional and online continuing nursing education, and the development of orientation of both professional and para-professional staff. She is a founding member of the National Nursing

Staff Development Organization and is a member of the editorial board of *Journal for Nurses in Staff Development*.

Chris Metzger Wilson, MSN, RN-BC
Director, Clinical Education and Professional Development, VUH, Vanderbilt University Medical Center, Nashville, TN

With clinical, management and educational experiences in a variety of settings, Ms. Wilson in her current role addresses a wide variety of activities including oversight of clinical orientation processes, Magnet education processes, active involvement in nursing leader development and a variety of other key functions. She is active in her local NNSDO affiliate, serving as the current president.

Debra M. Wolf, PhD, MSN, RN, BSN
Associate Professor of Nursing, Slippery Rock University, Slippery Rock Pennsylvania

Dr. Wolf has 30 years experience in acute care nursing and in academic settings. In her current position as the Program Chair of the Healthcare Informatics Certification Program, she leads several courses in health-care informatics for the undergraduate students. As Adjunct Faculty for Robert Morris University, Dr. Wolf leads DNP students in evidence-based practice and information systems technology. A member of several professional organizations, Dr. Wolf has served as mentor and coach for various nursing professionals.

Vanessa Worsham, MSN, APRN, ACNS-BC
Major, Army Nurse Corps, United States of America

A U.S. Army Nurse Corps Officer, MAJ Worsham is licensed as an Adult Clinical Nurse Specialist, Board-Certified. She has more than 13 years of management and clinical experience; Graduate Certificate in Business of Nursing from Johns Hopkins University and she is also a Certified Physical Fitness Specialist. She is a member of the NCLEX Examination Item Review and Development Panel. Her special clinical interests are advanced diabetes management and Transformational Leadership.

About the National Nursing Staff Development Organization

The National Nursing Staff Development Organization (NNSDO) advances the specialty practice of staff development for the enhancement of healthcare outcomes. Staff development as a specialty of nursing practice is defined by standards, based on research, and is critical to quality patient and organizational outcomes.

The purpose of NNSDO is to foster the art and science of nursing staff development, promote the image and professional status of nursing staff development, encourage and support nursing research and application of research findings in practice, and provide a platform for nurses engaged in staff development practice to discuss issues and make decisions related to the continuing evolution of the field of nursing staff development.

About the American Nurses Association

The American Nurses Association (ANA) is the only full-service professional organization representing the interests of the nation's 3.1 million registered nurses through its constituent member nurses associations, its organizational affiliates, and the Center for American Nurses. The ANA advances the nursing profession by fostering high standards of nursing practice, promoting the rights of nurses in the workplace, projecting a positive and realistic view of nursing, and by lobbying the Congress and regulatory agencies on health care issues affecting nurses and the public.

CONTENTS

Contributors   **iii**

**Scope and Standards of Nursing Professional Development
Practice**   **xi**
    Function of Scope of Practice Statement   xi
    Function of Standards   xi

Overview of Nursing Professional Development   **1**
    The Evolution of Nursing Professional Development (NPD)
      Practice   2
    Nursing Professional Development as Specialized Nursing Practice:
      A Systems Model   3
      Environment   4
      System Inputs   4
      System Throughputs   5
      System Outputs and Outcomes   7
      System Feedback   8

Scope of Practice for Nursing Professional Development   **9**
    Practice and Learning Environment   9
    Scope of Responsibility   10
    Educational Preparation and Qualifications of the NPD Specialist   12
      Education   12
      Certification   13
      Core Competencies   13
    Elements of Practice for the Nursing Professional Development
      Specialist   15
    Examples of Intertwined Elements of NPD Practice in
      Learning and Practice Environments   16
    Advocacy and Ethics   18
    Current and Future Issues, Innovations, and Trends   19

Standards of Nursing Professional Development Practice   **23**

Standards of Practice   **23**
Standard 1. Assessment   23

Standard   2. Identification of Issues and Trends   24
Standard   3. Outcomes Identification   25
Standard   4. Planning   26
Standard   5. Implementation   27
   Standard 5A. Coordination   28
   Standard 5B. Learning and Practice Environment 29
   Standard 5C. Consultation   30
Standard   6. Evaluation   31

Standards of Professional Performance for Nursing
Professional Development   **32**
Standard   7. Quality of NPD Practice   32
Standard   8. Education   33
Standard   9. Professional Practice Evaluation   34
Standard 10. Collegiality   35
Standard 11. Collaboration   36
Standard 12. Ethics   37
Standard 13. Advocacy   39
Standard 14. Research   40
Standard 15. Resource Utilization   41
Standard 16. Leadership   42

Glossary   **43**

References   **47**

Appendix A. Chronology of the Evolution of Nursing
Professional Development   **51**

Appendix B. *Scope and Standards for Professional Nursing*
***Development* (2000)**   **53**

Index   **95**

Scope and Standards of Nursing Professional Development Practice

Function of the Scope of Practice Statement

The scope of practice statement (pages 9–21) describes the "who", "what", "where", "when", "why" and "how" of nursing practice. Each of these questions must be sufficiently answered to provide a complete picture of the practice and its boundaries and membership. The depth and breadth in which individual registered nurses engage in the total scope of nursing practice is dependent upon education, experience, role, and the population served.

Function of Standards

These Standards, which are comprised of the Standards of Practice (pages 23–31) and the Standards of Professional Performance (pages 32–42), are authoritative statements by which nurses practicing within the role, population, and specialty governed by this document—*Nursing Professional Development: Scope and Standards of Practice*—and describe the duties that they are expected to competently perform. The Standards published herein may be utilized as evidence of the legal standard of care governing nurses practicing within the role, population, and specialty governed by this document. The Standards are subject to change with the dynamics of the nursing profession and as new patterns of professional practice are developed and accepted by the nursing profession and the public. In addition, specific conditions and clinical circumstances may also affect the application of the Standards at a given time; e.g., during a natural disaster. The Standards are subject to formal, periodic review and revision.

The measurement criteria that appear below each Standard are not all-inclusive and do not establish the legal standard of care. Rather, the measurement criteria are specific, measurable elements that can be used by nursing professionals to measure professional performance. Nurses practicing within this particular role, population, and specialty can identify opportunities for development and improvement by evaluating performance on these elements.

Overview of Nursing Professional Development

Nursing professional development (NPD) is a vital phase of lifelong learning in which nurses engage to develop and maintain competence, enhance professional nursing practice, and support achievement of career goals (ANA, 2000). Nursing professional development practice is a specialty that facilitates the lifelong learning and development activities of nurses aimed at influencing the actualization of professional growth and role competence and proficiency. Based on the sciences of nursing practice, learning, and change, NPD specialists use knowledge and skills in education theory and application, career development, leadership, and program management to support lifelong nursing professional development.

Building on a strong past (ANA, 1974, 1984, 1990, 1994, 2000 and as outlined in Appendix B), this revision of the scope and standards of practice for nursing professional development reflects the complex and rapidly developing factors that influence its current and future practice: globalization, dynamic practice environments, evidence-based practice, and the technologies of nursing and health care. Several changes are evident in this revision:

- An intentional focus on as a practice specialty, with less emphasis on the individual nurse's professional development;
- A new nursing professional development framework that more accurately portrays current and future NPD practice;
- A merging of roles and elements of practice that reflects changes in professional expectations;
- The operationalization of increased use of technology throughout healthcare environments; and
- The integration of evidence-based practice (EBP) and practice-based evidence (PBE).

This revision also reflects that nursing professional development practice varies depending on the knowledge and experience of the individual specialist and the scope of the practice setting. Accordingly, the specialty is addressed from a broad, deep perspective, which is grounded on the understanding that specialists will operationalize their NPD role based on their specific position within a particular setting while practicing within the defined scope and standards. The goal of this new edition is to create a dynamic trajectory for the future of nursing professional development.

The Evolution of Nursing Professional Development Practice

The past editions of the published scope and standards for nursing professional development practice have conceptualized this practice specialty by three overlapping domains:

- Staff development
- Continuing education
- Academia

A major evolution in nursing professional development practice, however, has been underway during the 10 years since the last edition. Within the continuing education and academic domains, technology has changed the learning environment and the potential target audiences. Once locally or regionally defined, the target audience is now global.

New methods of teaching and learning have developed, requiring changes in NPD specialist knowledge and expertise to develop programs using the new methods. The global market has created additional regulations and expectations to maintain the integrity and quality of educational programs. The dissemination and use of evidence-based practices has created a major change in academic and continuing education content. Yet, the purpose of nursing professional development remains to augment the knowledge, skills, and attitudes of nurses in their pursuit of professional career goals. Ultimately, this will enrich nursing's contributions to quality health care in order to protect the public.

The most profound transformation of nursing professional development practice has been within the staff development domain. This change may be due in part to a rapidly changing practice environment. The need for NPD specialists to use their expertise in assessment, planning, development, implementation, and evaluation to create change and promote quality has been recognized in the practice environment. Yet the change may be more reflective of the increasing levels of education and expertise of nurses practicing in staff development as has been set forward in past editions of the scope and standards. Due to growing knowledge and skills, NPD specialists are involved in program/project management, competency assessment, measurement, evaluation/return on investment, implementation of evidence-based practice, and development and coordination of excellence initiatives, all designed to enhance performance and professional development. As a result of the evolution of NPD specialty practice, a new model, the Nursing Professional Development Systems Model, has been created to capture current practice and accommodate future changes.

Nursing Professional Development as Specialized Nursing Practice: A Systems Model

Nursing professional development is a specialized nursing practice that facilitates the professional development of nurses in their participation in lifelong learning activities to enhance their professional competence and role performance, the ultimate outcomes of which are protection of the public and the provision of safe, quality care. The NPD process is best illustrated with a systems model consisting of interrelated inputs, throughputs, outputs, and feedback, as diagrammed in Figure 1.

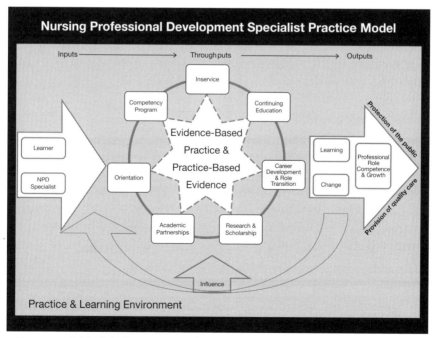

Figure 1. A Model of Nursing Professional Development Specialist Practice

Environment

The NPD specialist and the learner operate in two environments that have fluid and evolving boundaries. The nursing professional development practice environment may overlap with the learner's environment.

The NPD practice environment is the structural, social, and cultural setting in which nursing occurs. Multidimensional and subject to local, state, regional, national, and international regulations, initiatives, and trends, it creates ta context that influences practice behaviors and outcomes. The nursing professional development system is dependent on the material and human resources that exist within the practice environment. The NPD specialist enhances the practice environment through the promotion of transformational leadership and support of nursing's collaborative relationships with other disciplines and academic partnerships.

The learning environment is any context in which learning occurs. This environment may overlap with the practice environment. It is not limited to a physical classroom but includes alternate settings, including virtual ones.

System Inputs

Both the learner and the NPD specialist are seen as inputs that interface to contribute to the nursing professional development processes and overall success of the system.

Nursing Professional Development Specialist

The NPD specialist is a registered nurse with expertise in nursing education who influences professional role competence and professional growth of nurses in a variety of settings. The NPD specialist supports lifelong learners in an environment that facilitates continuous learning for nurses and other healthcare personnel. The NPD specialist fosters an appropriate climate for learning and facilitates the adult learning process.

Learner

The learner is an individual or group with an educational need who participates in professional development activities.

System Throughputs

A number of developmental and educational processes that revolve around evidence-based practice and practice-based evidence combine to contribute to the professional growth of practicing nurses and other learners. NPD specialists facilitate these processes based on the inputs. As inputs vary, so will the throughputs.

Evidence-Based Practice and Practice-Based Evidence

Evidence-based practice and practice-based evidence form the core of the nursing professional development model. EBP is the integration of the best research evidence, educational and clinical expertise, and learner values to facilitate decision-making (Sackett, Straus, Richardson, Rosenberg, & Haynes, 2000). NPD specialists use this science-to-service model of critical thinking to apply scientific knowledge such as research, scientific principles, and theory related to both educational methods and practice.

Complementary to EBP, practice-based evidence is a study methodology related more directly to practice effectiveness and improvement. The goal of PBE is to determine practices and interventions that work under normal day-to-day practice in terms of who, when, and at what cost (Horn & Gassaway, 2007). PBE studies allow a more in-depth understanding of individual variation and group differences (Evans, Connell, Barkham, Marshall, & Mellor-Clark, 2003). The NPD specialist uses this practice-to-science model to determine the most effective practice within a given context or group.

Orientation

Orientation is the educational process of introducing individuals who are new to the organization or department to the philosophy, goals, policies, procedures, role expectations, and other factors needed to function in a specific work setting. Orientation also takes place when changes in roles, responsibilities, and practice settings occur (ANA, 2000). The NPD specialist may develop, coordinate, administer, facilitate, conduct, and evaluate orientation programs for nursing and other healthcare personnel.

Competency Program

A competency is "an expected level of performance that integrates knowledge, skills, abilities, and judgment" (ANA, 2008, p. 3). A competency program is a group of activities designed to support an ongoing dynamic process of assessment and evaluation of performance. Competence is measured by "using tools that capture objective and subjective data about the individual's knowledge base and actual performance and are appropriate for the specific situation and the desired outcome…" (ANA, 2008, p. 6). The NPD specialist has expertise in competency assessment and may develop, coordinate, administer, facilitate, conduct, and evaluate competency programs.

In-service Education

In-service educational activities are those learning experiences designed in the work setting to assist individuals to acquire, maintain, and/or increase their ability to perform job functions within a given agency or institution (ANA, 2000). In-service activities include such things as policy and procedure changes and implementation of new products. The NPD specialist may develop, coordinate, administer, facilitate, conduct, and evaluate in-service education for nursing and other healthcare personnel.

Continuing Education

Continuing education refers to those systematic professional learning experiences designed to augment the knowledge, skills, and attitudes of nurses, thereby enriching the nurses' contributions to quality health care and their pursuit of professional career goals (ANA, 2000). The three different types of continuing education activities are *provider directed*, *learner directed*, and *learner paced* (ANCC, 2009a). Nurses apply knowledge gained from these activities to their practice, regardless of employer. The NPD specialist may create, manage, implement, coordinate, and evaluate continuing education.

Career Development and Role Transition

Career development involves identification and development of strategies that meet the career goals, tasks, and challenges in different stages throughout a nurse's career (Chang, Chou, & Cheng, 2006). The NPD specialist may assist others in their career development, role transition, and succession planning. NPD specialists may counsel others and coordinate, facilitate, conduct, and evaluate activities that promote career development and role transition.

Research and Scholarship

Participation in research and/or scholarly activities is highly dependent on the practice environment and role preparation of the NPD specialist. Nursing research is the use of systematic inquiry to develop or refine knowledge (Polit & Beck, 2008).

Scholarship is "application of the scientific process, which involves curiosity about what works and what does not, rigorous examination through both quantitative and qualitative approaches, peer review of the results, and their public dissemination" (Emerson & Records, 2008).

NPD specialists may conduct, encourage, disseminate, and/or participate in research and scholarship, including oral and poster presentations and publications (Bruce, 2009).

Academic Partnerships

Academic partnerships are mutually beneficial relationships between nursing schools and healthcare facilities. The partnerships represent a commitment between colleges/schools of nursing and healthcare facilities to support an environment of nursing development and continuous learning. Within the partnerships, NPD specialists may serve as academic liaisons, and they may teach, coordinate, and/or advise nurses and other learners concerning academic education and scholarly activity.

System Outputs and Outcomes

The overall outcome of nursing professional development is the acquisition of knowledge, skills, and attitudes that support safety and contribute to the *protection of the public and provision of quality care*. This is achieved by the following outputs of the system:

Change

Change is a movement to a desired state that subsequently becomes the basis for further transition (Sullivan & Decker, 2009). Change is reflected by adoption of new behaviors and/or processes.

Learning

Learning is the acquisition of knowledge, skills, abilities, and attitudes upon which to base practice. Learning is influenced by various factors such as individual characteristics, perceived needs, and teaching methodology.

Professional Role Competence and Growth

Professional role competence is performance that meets defined criteria based on the specialty area, context, and model of practice in which an individual nurse is engaged (ANA, 2008). Professional growth is defined as advancement through Benner's stages of clinical competence or progression in an organizational hierarchy (Benner 1984, 2001). One measure of professional role competence and growth is specialty certification. Specialty certification "validates nurses' skills, knowledge, and abilities ... within their professional sphere of activity and contributes to better patient outcomes" (ANCC, n.d.). NPD specialists pursue certification as practice educators while promoting certification of professional nurses in their respective nursing specialty.

System Feedback

The feedback loops represent the continuous lifelong learning and growth that influences the constantly evolving practice of nursing and nursing professional development. In this model, such *influence* (shown along the bottom of the diagram in Figure 1) in all its aspects is the process of affecting change, behaviors, and decisions of others. NPD specialists influence change by employing skills and knowledge to design and implement programs that produce desired outcomes. The NPD specialist influences decisions of others by using credible data, technology, relevant information, and documented outcomes within the learning and practice environment to shape both the system inputs and throughputs.

Scope of Practice for Nursing Professional Development

The scope of practice for the nursing professional development (NPD) specialist continues to evolve in support of changing roles in health care. This scope statement defines the who, what, where, when, why, and how of educational and learner needs that drive nursing professional development practice. Today the role of the NPD specialist is to address the learning needs of diverse groups through creativity, commitment, passion, and a high level of competence. As governing bodies, regulations, health policy, and consumer awareness continue to evolve, so do the expectations, requirements, demands, and responsibilities of the NPD specialist, thus requiring the scope of practice to broaden. The following content defines the various dimensions of the scope of practice within various healthcare arenas.

Practice and Learning Environment

The ultimate goal of nursing professional development practice is to support the provision of quality health care within local or global practice environments. This includes protecting the public by planning and implementing strategies that promote optimal learning and the effective translation of skills and knowledge to the learner's practice environment, thus enhancing their competence. The NPD specialist operates concurrently in two environments:

- *The practice environment*, which supplies resources and creates the context that influences practice behaviors and outcomes
- *The learning environment*, which is any context in which learning occurs.

These two environments have fluid and evolving boundaries. It is important to note that the two environments may intertwine at times to ensure successful learner and organizational outcomes. Examples of these environments may include, but are not limited to:

- Practice environments – Found in the following settings:
  - Hospitals
  - Long-term care facilities

- Academic institutions
- Public health facilities
- Outpatient/ambulatory clinics
- Community-clinic settings, including but not limited to home health settings and virtual health systems
- Any other setting where NPD specialists support quality outcomes
- Learning environments – Found in the following situations:
  - Virtual environments
  - Independent self-directed learning environments
  - Simulation labs
  - Practice environments
  - Classrooms
  - Academic settings
  - Conference, seminar, and workshop settings

Scope of Responsibility

The scope of responsibility and accountability for the NPD specialist continuously evolves to meet the demands of the practice setting. The following responsibilities may also vary based on environment and type of NPD specialist position description.

Career Development Responsibilities
- Career coaching
- Creating/supporting clinical advancement models
- Academic education coaching
- Assisting in role transition
- Planning for succession

Education Responsibilities
- Participating in continuing education
- Assessing and validating competency

- Coordinating student affiliations
- Assessing educational needs
- Participating in in-service activities
- Orienting
- Developing curricula

Leadership Responsibilities
- Collaborator at local, regional, state, national, and international levels to improve NPD practice
- Consultant
- Change agent/facilitator
- Encourager of shared governance
- Influencer of others for positive change
- Leader at various levels of the organization—group, department, system
- Facilitator of peer review/evaluations
- Preceptor, mentor, clinical coach, role model
- Facilitator of clinical/academic partnerships

Program Management Responsibilities
- Change agent facilitator
- Analyzer of data (gathering, interpreting, integrating)
- Overseer of evidence-based practice/practice-based evidence
- Facilitator of excellence initiatives (e.g., Magnet™, Baldridge)
- Preceptor, mentor, clinical coach
- Program consultant
- Planner, implementer, facilitator, and evaluator
- Program innovator (e.g., e-learning, simulation, etc.)
- Recordkeeper, reporter, and documenter of related material
- Manager and supporter of research initiatives

Compliance Initiative Responsibilities
- Government regulations
- Facility accreditation
- Licensure and nursing professional standards
- Other regulatory standards

Educational Preparation and Qualifications of the NPD Specialist

Like all registered nurses, completion of a degree program is the beginning of the career-long path that is professional development for an NPD specialist, which is validated through national certification and regularly updated. Specific core competencies are part of such formal validation of this specialty's knowledge and evaluation of a nurse's competency in the specialty practice.

Education

The NPD specialist is a licensed registered nurse with a graduate degree. If the graduate degree is in a related discipline, then the baccalaureate degree must be in nursing. Nurses working in nursing professional development are expected to demonstrate ongoing development of nursing professional development knowledge through continuing education, academic progression, and other professional development activities such as certification. All nurses working in this specialty , regardless of academic preparation, are expected to demonstrate the application of the standards of practice and professional performance for nursing professional development.

Due to the escalating complexity of nursing and the healthcare environment, the executive leader for nursing professional development should be a registered nurse, ideally prepared at the doctoral level in nursing or education. This recommendation clearly reflects the elevation of expectations for leadership in the area of professional development. Minimally, the administrator of the department should have a master's degree in nursing or related field. The educational and management expertise of the administrator is developed, maintained, and enhanced through self-evaluation and ongoing professional development activities.

Educators should demonstrate knowledge of appropriate methods of delivery of information and the ability to develop and facilitate relevant and effective education for adult learners. Other important skills of the NPD specialist that promote professional growth and self-actualization of the learner include mentoring and fostering empowerment. NPD specialists continue to evolve as professionals through their own self-assessment, ongoing development, and periodic self-evaluation.

Certification

Lifelong learning is important to develop and maintain competence and grow personally and professionally. National certification validates continuing professional development of the NPD specialist. Initial national certification is obtained through the successful completion of the certification examination in Nursing Professional Development through the American Nurses Credentialing Center (ANCC). Other certifications such as Nursing Education [NLN's Certified Nurse Educator (CNE)], Informatics, Clinical Nurse Specialist, Advanced Diabetes Management, etc., may complement and enhance the role of the NPD specialist. Specialty certification is renewed at regular intervals.

Core Competencies

The competencies listed below are to be considered as integral and core components of the NPD specialist role and are useful for validating specialists' knowledge and evaluating their competency (Brunt, 2007).

Career Development

- Accepts personal responsibilities for own professional development
- Promotes participation in professional organizations for self and others
- Demonstrates effective oral and written communication
- Uses effective interpersonal skills
- Fosters critical thinking
- Links nurses to professional development and other relevant resources

Education

- Assesses learner characteristics, including learning styles and learning needs for program development
- Creates an effective learning environment
- Demonstrates proficiency in use of technology
- Evaluates the outcomes of staff education
- Functions in the roles of both teacher and facilitator
- Implements a variety of teaching strategies tailored to the learners' characteristics, learning needs, cultural perspectives, and outcome objectives
- Plans NPD programs that are culturally relevant and that incorporate concepts of multicultural and multigenerational education
- Applies nursing and learning theoretical and conceptual foundations as a basis for developing NPD programs

Leadership

- Adheres to regulatory body/agency standards
- Advocates for NPD programs that support the needs of the learner and the organization
- Anticipates and forecasts trends
- Demonstrates a sensitivity to ethical, cultural, and spiritual inclusion
- Engages in ethical decision-making
- Effectively facilitates group processes
- Follows regulatory requirements for health reporting
- Functions as a change agent and leader
- Implements motivational strategies at the individual, group, program, and organizational levels
- Maintains confidentiality of sensitive information
- Uses outcome measurements and outcome evaluation methods
- Promotes problem solving
- Interprets and uses research in practice

- Demonstrates knowledge of the research process
- Models the application of evidence-based practice
- Uses organizational strategic plan and goals to determine educational priorities
- Develops financial plan that allocates resources to support NPD

Program and Project Management
- Plans and implements programs and projects, using innovation and creativity
- Consistently uses planning methodologies when implementing, facilitating, and evaluating various programs and projects
- Designs and implements evaluation plans for programs and projects
- Develops and implements a budget for programs and/or projects

Elements of Practice for the Nursing Professional Development Specialist

In the original edition, *Scope and Standards of Nursing Professional Development* (ANA, 2000), six roles were identified: educator, facilitator, change agent, consultant, leader, researcher. While these roles remain elements of the practice of the professional development nurse, they are no longer separate roles but are intertwined as the complexity of nursing professional development practice increases.

NPD specialists are engaged in a variety of ever-evolving healthcare arenas within our society. Today culture, technology, and collaboration in health care impact the elements of practice on an international level. The NPD specialist must be aware of and embrace the differences and commonalities within our professional practice, health care, and society. The practitioner must take a leading role in the change process by embracing and guiding change.

Accordingly, nursing professional development has significantly changed and expanded as knowledge of the learning process and technology has evolved.

The learning process begins by assessing the needs of the learners and ensuring that adult learning principles are incorporated. The NPD specialist collaborates with stakeholders to identify desired outcomes. The learning objectives are derived from the desired outcomes.

The delivery methods are evaluated, and the most appropriate are selected. Methods may include, but are not limited to, live presentations, self-learning packets, structured academic courses, and web-based courses. Qualified individuals such as the NPD specialist, nursing instructors, and academic faculty members are selected to plan and develop the learning experience. Thereafter, the NPD specialist plans, develops, and implements educational activities to foster the development of competence in the learner.

Upon completion of a learning experience, an evaluation measures the attainment of objectives and compares desired to actual outcomes. This evaluation process helps guide the restructuring and planning for future learning.

The NPD specialist needs a strong knowledge base in teaching and learning theories; curriculum design; methods for validation of learning; research processes; and innovative technological options. Collaboration between the learner and the NPD specialist enables the learner to document achievements, develop an awareness of self-perspective, and enrich his/her own professional practice. NPD specialists use innovative technologies and strategies to strengthen critical thinking and problem-solving abilities of the learner. The elements of practice, outlined below, are enlisted to assist the learner on the journey of professionalism.

Examples of Intertwined Elements of NPD Practice in Learning and Practice Environments

The NPD specialist may practice in a variety of organizational and entrepreneurial endeavors. The mission, vision, and goals of an organization are a guide for the NPD specialist's priorities and goals. NPD specialists practice with an awareness of who, what, and how specific groups impact educational endeavors. The following are examples of intertwined elements of nursing professional development practice.

Educator/Facilitator

- Develop an assessment process to determine learning needs
- Facilitate the adult learning process and actively involve the learner

- Assist in the selection of the most appropriate method of teaching to accommodate learning styles and the learning environment
- Enlist qualified instructors to plan, develop, and present material
- Evaluate outcomes
- Restructure program or educational plan as needed for future endeavors
- Develop and maintain a level of competency appropriate to one's practice environment or area of expertise
- Acquire identified resources needed for quality program design and delivery

Educator/Academic Liaison

- Mentor peers or colleagues
- Manage academic relations
- Serve as preceptor
- Collaborate with academia to advance curricula to meet the needs of healthcare organizations and the profession
- Provide supportive educational resources or opportunities

Change Agent/Team Member

- Compare and contrast healthcare issues and systematically analyze for needed change related to educational support
- Incorporate changes into learning activities
- Support organizations as they implement change
- Collaborate with intraprofessional and interprofessional groups
- Facilitate team building
- Problem solve where identified changes are needed

Researcher/Consultant

- Participate in and incorporate research and/or evidence-based practice as an advisor, investigator, collaborator, translator, integrator, or evaluator

- Incorporate research and/or evidence-based learning into educational activities and practice
- Serve as a resource to individuals, groups, and organizations to identify issues and possible internal and external resources

Leader/Communicator

- Provide support and direction to carry out organizational goals
- Promote nursing professional development as a practice specialty
- Use effective communication skills
- Demonstrate leadership on a professional level, maintaining appropriate competencies and involvement in activities at community, state, national, or international levels
- Influence change processes
- Integrate ethical principles in all aspects of practice

Collaborator/Advisor/Mentor

- Support lifelong learning in collaboration with academic institutions, healthcare organizations, professional nursing organizations, and other NPD specialists
- Support lifelong learning by advising/mentoring nurses as they execute a professional development plan
- Model professionalism and integrity

As the practice of nursing changes, the elements of practice for the NPD specialist also change. An example of this is the increasing use of evidence- based practice and research within nursing. The roles, responsibilities, and accountabilities of NPD specialists by necessity will change and continue changing, and as practitioners they must embrace and take a leading role in the process.

Advocacy and Ethics

Advocacy and adherence to ethical principles are essential components of NPD practice. The American Nurses Association (2008) considers health care as a universal right, transcending all individual differences. Within every healthcare community, cultural competence has emerged as a goal, due to the increasing cultural and religious diversity in our society. The NPD specialist demonstrates valuing diversity by providing programs and processes that support an array of ethical, cultural, educational, and diverse needs of patients and clinical professionals. The NPD specialist guides individual learners toward a global view of health care through both educational and self-reflective means.

Today's workforce is culturally diverse and multigenerational. NPD specialists advocate, support, and integrate appropriate methodology and resources for all types of learners' individual needs. The NPD specialist integrates ethical principles as outlined by the ANA Code of Ethics for Nurses (ANA, 2001) in all aspects of practice. Advances in healthcare technology and science, increasingly diverse patient populations, and social and legal issues lead to ethical dilemmas for the healthcare provider. The NPD specialist advocates for nursing ethics and often functions as a role model. As an advocate for the learner, the NPD specialist uses educational principles, standards, and methodologies to protect the autonomy, dignity, and rights of all individuals involved in the learning process. The NPD specialist promotes learning in a nonjudgmental and nondiscriminatory manner that is supportive of the diversity of the learners.

As part of their ethical responsibilities, NPD specialists must incorporate and respect the codes of ethics of other professionals, which may impact the processes used by nursing. An example of another profession's code of ethics is the Pharmaceutical Research and Manufacturers of America's *Code on Interactions with Healthcare Professionals* (PhRMA 2009). This organization represents research-based pharmaceutical and biotechnology companies. As a result of reviewing and incorporating this and other professions' codes of ethics, NPD specialists have demonstrated their awareness of restrictions regarding support.

Confidentiality is important as the NPD specialist promotes learning opportunities, collects data, and completes competency assessments. Rights, responsibilities, and accountability regarding confidential information are included in the education of the learner. Educational opportunities provided by the NPD specialist are presented without bias or conflict of interest in order to maintain ethical practice.

Current and Future Issues, Innovations, and Trends

Care has been taken to ensure that this edition reflects the trends and potential opportunities projected for the future. Current and future trends indicate that health care is in a dynamic state and is predicted to remain so well into the future. This state of constant evolution will place NPD specialists in the pivotal role of helping their organization and the staff they serve to adapt to the demands of this change. In this process, the NPD specialist must remain flexible and maintain a future focus, proactively leading change rather than reacting to emerging trends. As the specialty continues to advance, support from international, national, state, and local nursing organizations and health policy makers, as well as state and federal officials, are resources to further strengthen the influence of the NPD specialist. Among the projected are the following:

Workforce
- Generational issues influencing how people work together in the healthcare setting
- Evolving science of adult learning and developmental needs, including the "emerging adult" (Tanner, Arnett, & Leis, 2009)
- Knowledge management strategies needed for personnel as they exit the workforce
- Further diversification of the workforce
- Progressive education expectations for nurses at all levels
- Continued need for succession planning
- Increased integration of technology throughout the workforce
- Growing shortages of healthcare professionals

Clinical Practice
- New knowledge integrated into the practice setting
- Progressive education expectations for nurses at all levels
- Increasing advances of technology in care settings
- Developments in genetics and genomics
- Continued focus on quality outcomes, competency, and patient safety in healthcare settings
- Patient populations with more complex clinical needs associated with the impact of chronic illnesses, aging, and greater cultural diversity

- Increased demands for clinical placements of students
- Greater need for innovative partnerships between practice and education

Professional Development Practice
- Potential for educational strategies that can address the learning needs of individual, whether at the national or global level
- Incorporation of findings of research and evidence-based learning strategies (for example, cognitive research in the context of the physiology of learning)
- Considerations for retooling the workforce to enhance competencies to care for diverse patient populations with more complex clinical needs
- Greater emphasis on the use of technology to facilitate learning, such as simulation, distance, and web-based learning
- Need to develop strategies that promote rapid learning
- Focus on transition of newly graduated nurses into practice
- Growing need for succession planning for future nurse leaders
- Increased emphasis on demonstrating return on investment (ROI) of nursing professional development/education, necessitating the possession of greater business acumen by those in staff development
- Increased number of acute care settings, organizations, and agencies that have been approved as continuing nursing education providers by such organizations as the American Nurses Credentialing Center or ANA's constituent member associations

Organizational
- Increasingly complex healthcare systems due to mergers, acquisitions, and expansions
- Challenges in presenting learning as an investment in human capital and cost avoidance versus an expenditure
- Continued challenges in healthcare funding and reimbursements

STANDARDS OF NURSING PROFESSIONAL DEVELOPMENT PRACTICE

STANDARD 1. ASSESSMENT
The nursing professional development specialist collects data and information related to educational needs and other pertinent situations.

Measurement Criteria

The NPD specialist:

- Oversees the systematic and purposeful collection of data, information, and knowledge.

- Collects data from a variety of sources including, but not limited to, the nurse and the interdisciplinary healthcare team, professional organizations, consumers, healthcare experts, reports on health-related trends, key stakeholders, and legislative venues.

- Prioritizes data-collection activities based on the immediate or anticipated needs of the situation.

- Uses current technologies to facilitate comprehensive assessment of individual and organizational needs.

- Collects pertinent data using valid and reliable techniques and instruments including, but not limited to, focus groups, questionnaires, evaluations of past programs, and analysis of trends.

- Uses developmentally appropriate and evidence-based assessment techniques or instruments to define potential issues, problems, and needs.

- Uses analytical models and assessment tools that facilitate problem solving.

- Synthesizes available data, information, and knowledge relevant to the situation to identify patterns and variances.

- Documents relevant data in a retrievable format.

- Sustains an ongoing process for data collection.

STANDARD 2. IDENTIFICATION OF ISSUES AND TRENDS

The nursing professional development specialist analyzes issues, trends, and supporting data to determine the needs of individuals, organizations, and communities.

Measurement Criteria

The NPD specialist:

- Derives target audience needs and abilities from the assessment data.

- Validates identified needs with the nurse, consumer, content experts, and other educators or disciplines when possible and appropriate.

- Prioritizes individual and agency needs and addresses them in a timely manner.

- Uses data to identify future trends and issues.

- Documents identified needs in a manner that facilitates generation of purpose statements, educational objectives, program content, and evaluation criteria.

Standard **3.** Outcomes Identification
The nursing professional development specialist identifies desired outcomes.

Measurement Criteria

The NPD specialist:

- Involves learners and key stakeholders in formulating desired outcomes.

- Develops outcomes that reflect professional role competence, learning, and change.

- Develops context-specific outcomes based on: organizational, stakeholders', and learners' values and goals; and current evidence and regulations.

- Revises outcomes based on changes in trends, evidence, or stakeholders' expectations.

- Uses outcomes to demonstrate that programs are meeting their intended purpose and quality.

- Documents outcomes, including those that demonstrate learning and program impact.

STANDARD 4. PLANNING
The nursing professional development specialist establishes a plan that prescribes strategies, alternatives, and resources to achieve expected outcomes.

Measurement Criteria

The NPD specialist:

- Individualizes content to the target audience (e.g., educational level, experience, and preferred method of learning), the resources available, and the domains of learning.

- Develops content in collaboration with representatives of the target audience and with content experts.

- Prepares content reflective of the stated objectives and evidence-based practice.

- Considers adult learning concepts and instructional design principles when planning an activity.

- Collaborates with other disciplines to enhance the comprehensiveness of the plan.

- Considers the economic impact of the learning activities and organizational changes.

- Markets the plan, using promotional materials that are accurate, comprehensive, and appeal to the target audience.

- Documents the planning process.

STANDARD 5. IMPLEMENTATION
The nursing professional development specialist implements the identified plan.

Measurement Criteria

The NPD specialist:

- Implements the plan in a safe and timely manner.
- Uses evidence-based knowledge specific to the issue or trend to achieve the defined outcomes.
- Coordinates clinical, financial, technical, educational, and other resources and systems needed to implement the plan.
- Collaborates with colleagues and stakeholders.
- Implements the plan using principles and concepts of quality, project, or systems management.
- Engages organizational systems and resources that support implementation.
- Documents implementation and any modifications, including changes or omissions, of the identified plan.

STANDARD 5A. COORDINATION

The nursing professional development specialist coordinates educational initiatives and activities.

Measurement Criteria

The NPD specialist:

- Coordinates implementation of the plan, including activities and resources necessary to achieve desired outcomes.

- Coordinates human, financial, systems, and community resources necessary to implement the plan.

- Provides leadership in the coordination of multidisciplinary healthcare and community resources for integrated education and services.

- Documents coordination of the activities.

STANDARD 5B. LEARNING AND PRACTICE ENVIRONMENT
The nursing professional development specialist employs strategies and techniques to promote positive learning and practice environments.

Measurement Criteria

The NPD specialist:

- Promotes education of the learners to meet their professional development needs.

- Selects appropriate psychomotor, cognitive, and affective educational content, materials, techniques, and strategies for a positive learning environment.

- Uses educational strategies that are varied and designed to meet the needs of the learner.

- Integrates learning resources into systems that also address topics such as healthy lifestyles, risk-reducing behaviors, developmental needs, activities of daily living, and self care.

- Evaluates resources within the area of practice for accuracy, readability, and comprehensibility to help learners, patients, family, groups, or populations access quality information.

- Creates opportunities for feedback and evaluation of the effectiveness of the educational content, materials, techniques, strategies, and learning environment.

STANDARD 5C. CONSULTATION
The nursing professional development specialist provides consultation to influence plans, enhance the abilities of others, and effect change.

Measurement Criteria

The NPD specialist:

- Synthesizes data and information, while incorporating conceptual or theoretical frameworks, when providing consultation.

- Facilitates the effectiveness of a consultation by involving the learners, stakeholders, and members of other specialties in the decision-making process and negotiation of role responsibilities.

- Communicates consultation recommendations that influence the identified plan, facilitate understanding by stakeholders, enhance the work of others, and effect change.

- Establishes formal and informal consultative relationships that may lead to professional development or mentorship opportunities.

- Advises on the design, development, implementation, and evaluation of materials and teaching strategies appropriate to the situation and the learner's developmental level, learning needs, readiness, ability to learn, language preference, and culture.

- Considers theories pertaining to learning, behavioral change, motivation, epidemiology, and other related frameworks in consulting and collaborating when designing educational materials and programs.

- Develops recommendations and strategies to address problems and complex issues.

STANDARD 6. EVALUATION
The nursing professional development specialist evaluates progress toward attainment of outcomes.

Measurement Criteria

The NPD specialist:

- Selects valid, reliable, and relevant methods and instruments to measure processes and outcomes.

- Involves learners and stakeholders in the evaluation process.

- Implements a systematic and useful evaluation plan aimed at measuring processes and outcomes that are relevant to program, learners, and stakeholders.

- Documents the results of evaluation.

- Synthesizes evaluation data, trends, and expectations to guide decision-making about changes and improvement of all components of NPD practice.

- Revises programs based on evaluation data.

- Disseminates the evaluation results of learning activities and educational programs.

STANDARDS OF PROFESSIONAL PERFORMANCE FOR NURSING PROFESSIONAL DEVELOPMENT

STANDARD 7. QUALITY OF NURSING PROFESSIONAL DEVELOPMENT PRACTICE

The nursing professional development specialist systematically enhances the quality and effectiveness of nursing professional development practice.

Measurement Criteria

The NPD specialist:

- Applies the nursing process in a responsible, accountable, and ethical manner.

- Uses creativity and innovation to improve the quality of the learning experience.

- Uses current best evidence.

- Ensures the presence of effective mechanisms for the development, implementation, and evaluation of NPD practice.

- Incorporates new knowledge and skills to initiate change.

- Obtains or maintains professional certification.

- Participates in quality performance improvement activities.

- Participates in the evaluation and regulation of individuals as appropriate through privileging, credentialing, or certification processes.

- Documents the evaluation of nursing professional development activities.

STANDARD 8. EDUCATION
The nursing professional development specialist maintains current knowledge and competency in nursing and professional development practice.

Measurement Criteria

The NPD specialist:

- Participates in educational activities related to appropriate knowledge bases and professional issues.

- Acquires knowledge and skills appropriate to the specialty area, practice setting, role, and learner diversity.

- Seeks experiences to develop, maintain, and improve competence in nursing professional development.

- Uses self-reflection and inquiry to identify learning needs.

- Uses current research findings and other evidence to expand knowledge, enhance role performance, and increase knowledge of professional issues.

STANDARD 9. PROFESSIONAL PRACTICE EVALUATION

The nursing professional development specialist evaluates his/her own practice in relation to professional practice standards and guidelines, and relevant statutes, rules, and regulations.

Measurement Criteria

The NPD specialist:

- Participates in systematic peer review.

- Seeks feedback regarding his/her own practice from learners, professional partners, peers, and supervisors or other administrators, as appropriate.

- Examines application of current standards, guidelines, and relevant rules and regulations.

- Demonstrates respect for diversity by considering cultural, ethnic, generational, and other such differences in meeting learner needs.

- Interacts with peers and colleagues to enhance his/her own NPD practice and role performance.

- Evaluates his/her own performance on a regular basis, identifying areas of strength as well as areas in which professional development would be beneficial.

- Takes action to achieve goals identified during the professional practice evaluation process.

STANDARD 10. COLLEGIALITY
The nursing professional development specialist establishes collegial partnerships contributing to the professional development of peers, students, colleagues, and others.

Measurement Criteria

The NPD specialist:

- Shares knowledge and skills with peers and colleagues through activities such as presentations at meetings and professional conferences and by participation in professional organizations.

- Provides peers with feedback regarding their practice and role performance.

- Contributes to an environment that fosters ongoing educational experiences for colleagues, other healthcare professionals, and learners.

- Contributes to a supportive, healthy, and safe work environment that fosters mutual respect.

- Interacts with peers, students, colleagues, and others to enhance professional nursing, nursing professional development practice, and role performance of self and others.

- Models expert practice to peers, interprofessional team members, healthcare consumers, and learners.

STANDARD 11. COLLABORATION

The nursing professional development specialist collaborates with interprofessional teams, leaders, stakeholders, and others to facilitate nursing practice and positive outcomes for consumers.

Measurement Criteria

The NPD specialist:

- Communicates with healthcare providers and key stakeholders regarding educational programs and activities.

- Develops partnerships and coalitions with others to enhance health care through interprofessional activities such as education, consultations, program management, and administration.

- Partners with others to effect change and generate positive outcomes.

- Engages colleagues in the planning and implementation of lifelong learning activities for individuals and groups of learners.

- Documents plans and communications of collaborative endeavors.

Standard 12. Ethics
The nursing professional development specialist integrates ethics in all areas of practice.

Measurement Criteria

The NPD specialist:

- Incorporates *Code of Ethics for Nurses with Interpretive Statements* (ANA, 2001), *Nursing Professional Development: Scope and Standards of Practice,* and other relevant standards, guidelines, benchmarks, regulations, and laws to guide practice.

- Employs educational principles, standards, and methodologies in a manner that preserves and protects the autonomy, dignity, and rights of all individuals involved in the educational program and learning process.

- Employs educational principles, standards, and methodologies to establish and maintain confidentiality.

- Performs role in a nonjudgmental and nondiscriminatory manner that is sensitive to learner diversity.

- Evaluates factors related to privacy, security, and confidentiality in the use and handling of data, information, and knowledge related to educational programs.

- Establishes a process to identify and address ethical issues within the learning environment.

- Develops educational programs free of commercial bias in accordance with the guidelines of the ANCC Commission on Accreditation and the guidelines from health-related disciplines.

- Assures that educational program and activity planners and others who may influence educational content declare potential or actual conflict of interest and that those declarations are available to potential learners in advance.

- Maintains procedures for monitoring educational activities to screen for potential or actual unethical behavior, commercial bias, compromise of intellectual property rights, or conflict of interest.

Continued ▶

- Mentors peers and others when situations arise that create ethical conflicts.

- Reports behaviors that are illegal, incompetent, unethical, inconsistent with practice standards, or reflective of impaired practice.

- Documents that the requirements of the accrediting bodies are consistently followed, reporting relevant issues and information to the respective body.

STANDARD 13. ADVOCACY

The nursing professional development specialist advocates for the protection and rights of individuals, families, communities, populations, healthcare providers, nursing and other professions, institutions, and organizations.

Measurement Criteria

The NPD specialist:

- Serves as an advocate representing learners.

- Promotes opportunities for lifelong learning for self and others.

- Supports the involvement of individuals in their own professional development and learning processes.

- Educates learners and other stakeholders with regard to rights, responsibilities, and accountability involved in the collection, access, use, and exchange of protected information.

STANDARD 14. RESEARCH
The nursing professional development specialist integrates research findings into practice.

Measurement Criteria

The NPD specialist:

- Uses the best available evidence to guide practice decisions.

- Creates a supportive environment for nursing research, scholarly inquiry, generation of knowledge, and translation of research into practice.

- Supports research activities that align with the organizational strategic plan.

- Participates in research activities at various levels appropriate to the NPD specialist's education and role.

- Contributes to the development of lifelong learning and nursing professional development practice by supporting, conducting, and synthesizing research.

- Disseminates research findings through activities such as presentations, publications, consultation, educational programs, courses, activities, and use of other media.

STANDARD 15. RESOURCE UTILIZATION
The nursing professional development specialist considers factors related to safety, effectiveness, and cost in regard to professional development activities and expected outcomes.

Measurement Criteria

The NPD specialist:

- Evaluates factors such as safety, effectiveness, availability, cost and benefits, efficiencies, opportunities for learners, and impacts on practice.

- Allocates human, financial, and material resources based on identified needs and goals.

- Assists stakeholders in identifying and securing appropriate and available learning opportunities.

- Delegates tasks based on the knowledge, skills, and abilities of the individual, the complexity of the task, and the predictability of the outcome.

- Develops innovative solutions and strategies to secure appropriate resources and technology for professional development initiatives.

- Administers human resources, facilities, materials, equipment, and technologies for educational purposes.

- Establishes strategies to promote recognition of the role of professional development within the organization.

- Monitors resource allocation and utilization.

- Documents resource utilization decisions and activities.

STANDARD 16. LEADERSHIP
The nursing professional development specialist provides leadership in the professional practice setting and the profession.

Measurement Criteria

The NPD specialist:

- Works to create and maintain healthy work environments in educational and practice settings.

- Partners in setting goals to ensure that educational programs are aligned with organizational goals and strategic plan.

- Exhibits creativity and flexibility through times of change.

- Demonstrates energy, excitement, and a passion for quality work.

- Creates a practice culture in which innovation and risk taking are promoted and expected.

- Assumes leadership roles representing nursing professional development.

- Influences decision-making bodies to maintain and improve quality nursing and professional development programs.

- Promotes the professional development program mission, goals, action plans, and outcome measures.

- Provides guidance, resources, and knowledge for professional growth of others.

- Advances the profession through writing, publishing, presenting, and participating with professional interdisciplinary and multidisciplinary audiences, and through participating in nursing and professional development organizations.

- Demonstrates responsibility for reporting to licensing, certification, accreditation, and other regulatory bodies for educational program compliance.

- Mentors colleagues, other nurses, students, and others as appropriate.

Glossary

Academic partnerships. Mutually beneficial relationships between nursing schools and healthcare facilities.

Competency. "An expected level of performance that integrates knowledge, skills, abilities, and judgment" (ANA, 2008, p. 3).

Competency program. A group of activities designed to support an ongoing dynamic process of assessment and evaluation of performance.

Continuing education. Those systematic professional learning experiences designed to augment the knowledge, skills, and attitudes of nurses, and therefore enrich nurses' contributions to quality health care and to their pursuit of professional career goals (ANA, 2000).

Core competency. A defined fundamental level of knowledge, ability, skill, or expertise that is essential to a particular job.

Emerging adult. A person, typically age 18–29, who is in the development process of gaining self-sufficiency and learning to balance self-need, work responsibilities, and family. This is a time when learning is moving from social mandate to individual responsibility. The emerging adult focuses on applying acquired knowledge and practical problem solving skill in real-life situations.

Evidence-based practice (EBP). The integration of the best research evidence, educational and clinical expertise, and learner values to facilitate decision-making (Sackett et al., 2000).

In-service educational activities. Those learning experiences designed in the work setting to assist individuals to acquire, maintain, and/or increase their ability to perform job functions within a given agency or institution (ANA, 2000).

Interdisciplinary. The inclusion of two or more disciplines within health-related professions. The planners and/or the learners may be interdisciplinary as appropriate for the development and implementation of learning opportunities.

Interprofessional. The inclusion of two or more professions. It may include individuals, groups, and/or knowledge from other professions that are relevant for specific learning opportunities. An example would be including experts from the field of education when planning health-related in-service, staff development, or continuing education programs. Individuals or groups may be included from these other professions as members of the audience.

Learner. An individual or group with an educational need who participates in professional development activities.

Learner-directed. "A learning activity in which the learner takes the initiative, with or without the help of others, in diagnosing his/her learning needs, formulating learning goals, identifying human and material resources for learning, choosing and implementing appropriate learning strategies, and evaluating learning outcomes. Learner-directed activities may be developed with or without the help of others, but they are engaged in by only one individual" (ANCC, 2009).

Learner-paced. A continuing nursing education activity where the learner determines the pace at which he/she engages in the learning activity (ANCC, 2009).

Learning environment. Any context in which learning occurs.

Lifelong learning. The continual acquisition of knowledge and skills throughout life in preparation for and as a response to the different roles, situations, and environments encountered. Lifelong learning can occur in formal and informal education systems, both within and outside the workplace.

Mentor. A respected professional who serves as a role model, advisor, counselor, and confidant. Encourages and facilitates lifelong learning based upon a mutual attraction to learning (Bruce, 2009).

Nursing professional development (NPD) practice environment. The structural, social, and cultural setting in which nursing professional development occurs.

Nursing professional development (NPD) specialist. A registered nurse with expertise in nursing education who: influences professional role competence and professional growth of nurses in a variety of settings; supports lifelong learning of nurses and other healthcare personnel in an environment that facilitates continuous learning; and fosters an appropriate climate for learning and facilitates the adult learning process.

Orientation. The educational process of introducing individuals who are new to the organization or department to the philosophy, goals, policies, procedures, role expectations, and other factors needed to function in a specific work setting.

Partner. A mutually beneficial association between individuals with a common need, goal, activity, or sphere of interest.

Peer review. A collegial, systematic, and periodic process by which registered nurses are held accountable for practice and that fosters the refinement of one's knowledge, skills, and decision-making at all levels and in all areas of practice (ANA, 2004, p. 49).

Practice-based evidence (PBE). A study methodology related more directly to practice effectiveness and improvement and that promotes a greater understanding of individual and group differences (Evans et al., 2003).

Professional role competence. Performance that meets defined criteria based on the specialty area, context, and model of practice in which an individual nurse is engaged (ANA, 2008).

Provider-directed. "The provider controls all aspects of the learning. The provider determines the learning objectives based on needs assessments, content of the learning activity, the method by which it is presented and evaluation methods. Provider-directed activities may be presented in a number of different vehicles: electronic, journal, lecture, etc." (ANCC, 2009).

Outcome. Something that follows, is the result of, or is the consequence of a project, program, or event.

Outcome measurement. The process of observing, describing, and quantifying predefined indicators of outcomes of performance.

Outputs. The change that occurs to the input as the result of the process. In the NPD Specialist Practice Model, *outputs* reflect the learning, change, and professional role competence and growth of the learner and the NPD specialist.

Return on investment (ROI). The relative value of a program or project based on a cost and net-benefit ratio.

Simulation. An attempt to mimic essential aspects of a clinical situation with the goal of understanding and managing the situation better when it occurs in actual clinical practice. A technique that uses a situation or environment created to allow persons to experience a representation of a real event for the purpose of practice, learning, evaluation, testing, or to gain understanding of systems or human actions (Simulation Innovation Resource Center, 2009).

Succession planning. The formal process in which or the condition under which arrangements are predetermined for the continued intentional development of an individual within an organization or department.

Stakeholder. Any individual or group who has a vested interest in the product or outcome of a project, program, or organization.

Target audience. "Group for which an educational activity has been designed" (ANA, 2000, p. 26).

Transformational nursing leader. One who: leads in order to meet the demands of the future; creates the vision and provides the resources to achieve that vision; communicates need for change as well as each unit's role in the change process; requires "vision, influence, clinical knowledge, and a strong expertise relating to professional nursing practice" (ANCC, 2008).

REFERENCES

All URLs were active when retrieved on April 15, 2010.

American Nurses Association (ANA). (1974). *Standards for continuing education in nursing.* Kansas City, MO: American Nurses Publishing.

American Nurses Association (ANA). (1975). *Accreditation of continuing education in nursing.* Kansas City, MO: American Nurses Publishing.

American Nurses Association (ANA). (1976a). *Continuing education in nursing: An overview.* Kansas City, MO: American Nurses Publishing.

American Nurses Association (ANA). (1976b). *Guidelines for staff development.* Kansas City, MO: American Nurses Publishing.

American Nurses Association (ANA). (1978). *Self-directed continuing education in nursing.* Kansas City, MO: American Nurses Publishing.

American Nurses Association (ANA). (1984). *Standards for continuing education in nursing.* Kansas City, MO: American Nurses Publishing.

American Nurses Association (ANA). (1990). *Standards for nursing staff development.* Kansas City, MO: American Nurses Publishing.

American Nurses Association (ANA). (1992). *Roles and responsibilities for nursing continuing education and staff development across all settings.* Kansas City, MO: American Nurses Publishing.

American Nurses Association (ANA). (1994). *Standards for nursing professional development: Continuing education and staff development.* Washington, DC: American Nurses Publishing.

American Nurses Association (ANA). (2000). *Scope and standards of practice for nursing professional development.* Washington, DC: American Nurses Publishing.

American Nurses Association (ANA). (2001). *Code of ethics for nurses with interpretive statements*. Washington, DC: Nursesbooks.org.

American Nurses Association (ANA). (2004). *Nursing: Scope and standards of practice.*Silver Spring, MD: Nursesbooks.org.

American Nurses Association (ANA). (2008). Position statement, *Professional Role Competence.* http://www.nursingworld.org/NursingPractice

American Nurses Credentialing Center (ANCC). (2008). Announcing a New Model for ANCC's Magnet Recognition Program©. http://www.nurse-credentialing.org/Magnet/NewMagnetModel.aspx#Transformational Leadership

American Nurses Credentialing Center (ANCC). (2009). *Application manual: Accreditation program.* Silver Spring, MD: Author.

American Nurses Credentialing Center (ANCC). (n.d). *ANCC Nurse Certification.* Silver Spring, MD: Author. http://www.nursecredentialing.org/Certification.aspx

Benner, P.A. (1984). *From novice to expert: Excellence and power in clinical nursing practice*. Menlo Park, CA: Addison-Wesley.

Benner, P.A. (2001) *From novice to expert*: *Excellence and power in clinical nursing practice*. (Commemorative edition.) Upper Saddle River, NJ: Prentice Hall Health.

Bruce, S. (Ed.). (2009). *Core curriculum for nursing staff development* (3rd Edition). Pensacola, FL: National Nursing Staff Development Organization.

Brunt, B. (2007). *Competencies for staff educators*. Marblehead, MA: HCPro.

Chang, P., Chou, Y., & Cheng, F. (2006). Designing career development programs through understanding of nurses' career needs. *Journal for Nurses in Staff Development*, 246–253.

Emerson, R.J., & Records, K. (2008). Today's challenge, tomorrow's excellence: The practice of evidence-based education. *Journal of Nursing Education*, 47(8), 359–370.

Evans, C., Connell, J., Barkham, M., Marshall, C., & Mellor-Clark, J. (2003). Practice-based evidence: Benchmarking NHS primary care counseling services at national and local levels. *Journal of Clinical Psychology and Psychotherapy, 10,* 374–388.

Hemlinger, C. S. (1999) ANA creates new "house" for all nurses. *American Journal of Nursing*: 99(12), 59-60.

Horn, S.D., & Gassaway, J. (2007). Practice-based evidence study design for comparative effectiveness research. *Medical Care*, 45, S50–S57.

National Nursing Staff Development Organization. (NNSDO). (2009): *Core curriculum for nursing staff development*. (3rd ddition). Pensacola, FL: Author.

Pharmaceutical Research and Manufacturers of America (PhRMA). (2009). *Code on interactions with healthcare professionals*. Washington, DC: Author. http://www.phrma.org/code_on_interactions_with_healthcare_professionals

Polit, D., & Beck, C.T. (2008). *Nursing research: Generating and assessing evidence for nursing practice.* New York: Lippincott.

Sackett, D.L., Straus, S.E., Richardson, W.S., Rosenberg, W., & Haynes, R.B. (2000). *Evidence-based medicine: How to practice and teach EBM.* Edinburgh: Churchill Livingstone.

Simulation Innovation Resource Center (SIRC). (2009). National League for Nursing. *SIRC Glossary*. http://sirc.nln.org/mod/glossary/view.php?id=183

Sullivan, E.J., & Decker, P.J. (2009*). Effective leadership and management in nursing*, 7th edition. Upper Saddle River, NJ: Prentice Hall.

Tanner, J.I., Arnett, J.J., & Leis, J.A. (2009). Emerging adulthood: Learning and development during first stage of adulthood. In M.C. Smith & N. Defrates-Densch (Eds.). *Handbook of research on adult learning and development* (pp. 34–67). New York: Routledge.

APPENDIX A
CHRONOLOGY OF THE EVOLUTION OF NURSING PROFESSIONAL DEVELOPMENT

Adapted from ANA (2004), pp. 54–55.

1969   First national conference on nursing continuing education held in Williamsburg, VA, to provide a forum for discussion of national issues by college and university providers of nursing continuing education.

1972   Commission on Continuing Education is established by American Nurses Association.

1973   Article about Continuing Education Council membership published (Continuing Education Council seeks members, 1973).

1974   *Standards for Continuing Education in Nursing* published (ANA, 1974).

1975   *Accreditation of Continuing Education in Nursing* published (ANA, 1975).
        First members of the National Accreditation Board, the National Review committee, and five regional accrediting committees appointed by ANA's Commission on Nursing.

1976   *Continuing Education in Nursing: An Overview* (ANA, 1976a) published.
        Guidelines for Staff Development published (ANA, 1976b).

1978   *Self-Directed Continuing Education in Nursing* published (ANA, 1978).
        Guidelines for Staff Development revised. National workshops held to facilitate implementation in practice, which provided first recognition of evolving field of staff development in practice settings and its complement to nursing continuing education in academic settings.

1984   *Standards for Continuing Education in Nursing* published (ANA, 1984).

1989   Name for ANA Council on Continuing Education changed to Council on Continuing Education and Staff Development to reflect more clearly expansion of the field of specialty practice in nursing education.
National Nursing Staff Development Organization (NNSDO) established and incorporated.

1990   *Standards for Nursing Staff Development* published (ANA, 1990).

1991   American Nurses Credentialing Center (ANCC) established as a subsidiary of ANA to implement the credentialing programs, including certification for nurses and accreditation of continuing education.

1992   Certification in Nursing Continuing Education and Staff Development first offered by ANCC in collaboration with NNSDO.
Roles and Responsibilities for Nursing Continuing Education and Staff Development across All Settings published (ANA, 1992).

1994   *Standards for Nursing Professional Development: Continuing education and Staff Development* published (ANA, 1994).

1995   Name of the ANA Council changed to Council for Nursing Professional Education and Development.

1997   *Report of the ANA Council/NNSDO Task Force on Advanced Practice in Nursing Continuing Education and Staff Development* published.

1999   ANA Council for Nursing Professional Education and Development dissolved by action of ANA House of Delegates as part of revision to overall organizational structure (Hemlinger, 1999).

2000   *Scope and Standards of Practice for Nursing Professional Development* published (ANA, 2000).

2008   Position statement, *Professional Role Competence* published (ANA, 2008).

2009   *Core Curriculum for Nursing Staff Development* (3rd Edition) published (NNSDO, 2009).

2009   NNSDO's 20th anniversary in Philadelphia, PA, July 2009.

APPENDIX B
SCOPE AND STANDARDS OF PRACTICE FOR PROFESSIONAL NURSING DEVELOPMENT (2000)

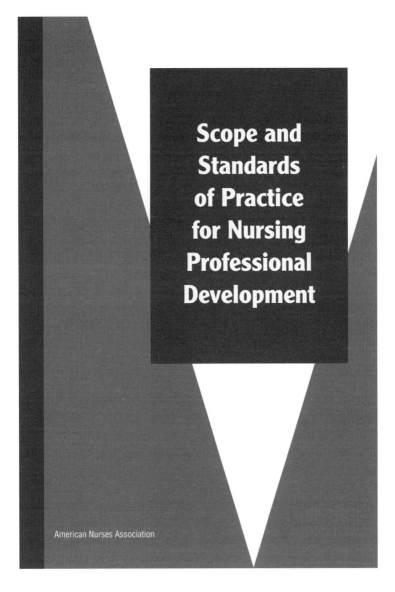

Scope and Standards of Practice for Nursing Professional Development

American Nurses Association

SCOPE and STANDARDS
of
Practice for Nursing Professional Development

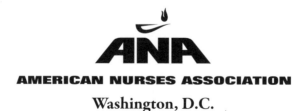

AMERICAN NURSES ASSOCIATION

Washington, D.C.

Library of Congress Cataloging-in-Publication Data

Scope and standards of practice for nursing professional development.
   p.   ; cm.
   Revision of: Standards for nursing professional development:
continuing education and staff development. 1994.
   Includes bibliographical references.
   1. Nursing—Study and teaching (Continuing education)—
Standards—United States. 2. Nurses—In-service training—
Standards—United States. 1. American Nurses' Association. II.
Standards for nursing professional development.
[DNLM: 1. Education, Nursing, Continuing—standards—United
States. 2. Nursing—standards—United States. 3. Staff Development—
standards—United States. WY 18.5 S422 2000]
RT76.S366 2000
610.73'071'55—dc21   00-042007

Published by
Nursesbooks.org
The Publishing Program of ANA
American Nurses Association
8515 Georgia Avenue, Suite 400
Silver Spring, MD 20910-3492

ISBN-13: 978-1-55810-237-8   ISBN-10: 1-55810-237-X

ACKNOWLEDGMENTS

Workgroup to Review and Revise Standards for Nursing Professional Development: Continuing Education and Staff Development

Mary Jane Ferrell, PhD, RN,C, Co-Chair
Gayle A. Pearson, DrPH, RN, Co-Chair
Dorothy Bell, MS, RN,C
RoAnne Dahlen-Hartfield, DNSc, RN
Nancy M. DiMauro, MA, RN,C
Alexia Green, PhD, RN
Barbara A. Brunt, MA, RN,C
Barbara Garrett, PhD, RN,C
Nancy Ridenour, PhD, RN

ANA Staff

Carol J. Bickford, MS, RN,C
Yvonne Humes, BBA
Winifred Carson, JD

This appendix is not current and is of historical significance only.

CONTENTS

Preface vii

Introduction 1
    Philosophy of Nursing Professional Development 1
    Framework for Nursing Professional Development 4

Scope of Practice for Nursing Professional Development 7
    Roles of Nursing Professional Development Educators ... 7
    Educational Preparation of Nursing Professional
        Development Educators 10

Standards of Practice for Nursing
Professional Development 12
    Standard I. Assessment 12
    Standard II. Diagnosis: Analysis to Determine Target
        Audience and Learner Needs 12
    Standard III. Identification of Educational Outcomes 13
    Standard IV. Planning 13
    Standard V. Implementation 14
    Standard VI. Evaluation 15

Standards of Professional Performance for
Nursing Professional Development 16
    Standard I. Quality of Nursing Professional
        Development Practice 16
    Standard II. Performance Appraisal 16
    Standard III. Education 17
    Standard IV. Collegiality 18
    Standard V. Ethics 18
    Standard VI. Collaboration 19
    Standard VII. Research 20
    Standard VIII. Management and Resource Utilization 21
    Standard IX. Leadership 22

Glossary 23

This appendix is not current and is of historical significance only.

Appendixes
A. Chronology of the Evolution of Nursing
   Professional Development 27
B. Chronology of American Nurses Association's
   Continuing Competence Initiatives 29
C. Responsibilities for Continuing Competence 31

References 33

PREFACE

Standards provide a means by which a profession clearly describes the focus of its activities, the recipients of service, and the responsibilities for which practitioners are accountable. As the professional organization for nursing, the American Nurses Association (ANA) has demonstrated a strong leadership role in the development, promotion, implementation, evaluation, and revision of standards since the mid 1960s (ANA 1965). ANA published the first standards of practice for the nursing profession in 1973, *Standards of Nursing Practice* (ANA 1973). These standards, in conjunction with the definition of the scope of nursing practice in *Nursing's Social Policy Statement* (ANA 1995) and the *Code for Nurses with Interpretive Statements* (ANA 1985), contribute to a definitive description and understanding of nursing's accountability to the public.

ANA first published the *Standards for Continuing Education in Nursing* in 1974 (ANA 1974) and the first *Standards for Nursing Staff Development* in 1990 (ANA 1990). See Appendix A for the chronology of the evolution of nursing professional development.

The *Scope and Standards of Practice for Nursing Professional Development* reflects a revision of the *Standards for Nursing Professional Development: Continuing Education and Staff Development* (ANA 1994) and incorporates the content included in the *Roles and Responsibilities for Nursing Continuing Education and Staff Development Across All Settings* (ANA 1992a). This document outlines the expectations of the full professional role within which nurses provide educational activities to those in the profession. The authority for the provision of these services is based on the social contract that acknowledges the professional rights, responsibilities, and public accountability addressed in *Nursing's Social Policy Statement* (ANA 1995) and the *Code for Nurses with Interpretive Statements* (ANA 1985).

This work supports the intent of the nursing profession to adhere to high standards in the delivery of educational programs by ensuring that qualified individuals provide nursing professional development and educational services. By assisting nurses in preparing for contemporary practice, nursing professional development educators ultimately contribute to improving the health and well-being of all individuals.

INTRODUCTION

Nursing professional development is the lifelong process of active participation by nurses in learning activities that assist in developing and maintaining their continuing competence, enhance their professional practice, and support achievement of their career goals. Nursing professional development begins within the basic nursing education program, continues throughout the career of the nurse, and encompasses the educational concepts of continuing education, staff development, and academic preparation.

This document defines the scope of practice, roles, and responsibilities for the specialty of nursing professional development and is consistent with the six standards of care and eight standards of professional performance for nurses (ANA 1998b). The standards of practice for nursing professional development include assessment, diagnosis, analysis to determine target audience and learner needs, identification of educational outcomes, planning, implementation, and evaluation. Standards of professional performance include quality of nursing professional development practice, performance appraisal, education, collegiality, ethics, collaboration, research, management and resource utilization, and leadership. The standards and corresponding outcome criteria focus on competencies appropriate for professional development educators practicing in all settings.

Philosophy of Nursing Professional Development

Beliefs

The following beliefs guided development of the *Scope and Standards of Practice for Professional Nursing Development*:

- Lifelong learning is the responsibility of the nurse and is essential to maintain and increase competence in nursing practice.

- Continuing professional nursing competence is essential to the provision of safe, quality health care to all members of society.

- The public has a right to expect continuing professional nursing competence throughout the career of the nurse.

- Assurance of continuing professional nursing competence must be shaped and guided by the nursing profession.

- Continuing professional nursing competence is definable, measurable, and can be evaluated.

- The nurse as the learner actively partners with the nursing professional development educator in the educational process and in the maintenance of the nurse's continuing professional nursing competence.

- The nursing professional development educator incorporates the roles of facilitator, change agent, consultant, leader, or researcher in the learning activities that support the nurse in developing and maintaining continuing professional nursing competence.

- Self-directed learning is an integral part of continuing education, staff development, and academic education.

- Use of adult learning principles contributes to effective professional development activities.

- A variety of educational options are necessary to meet the diverse needs of the nursing population, including, but not limited to, academic education, experiential learning, consultation, teaching others, professional reading, distance learning, research, and self-directed activities.

- The learning activity may be related to resolving the current knowledge or skill deficit of the nurse to ensure continuing professional nursing competence.

- Ongoing evaluation of educational activities is essential to maintain and enhance professional development and the quality and cost-effectiveness of health care.

- The practice of nursing professional development is guided by principles of ethics.

Influencing Factors

Professional development needs of nurses are influenced by many factors, such as

- Nurses' acceptance of accountability and responsibility for their practice.

- Specialization in nursing, cultural backgrounds, changes in educational levels, and other demographic characteristics of nursing adult learners.

- Changes in demographic characteristics of health care consumer populations.

- Knowledgeable consumers who recognize their right to health care and demand accountability for services rendered.

- Changing health care delivery systems and financing methods.

- A rapidly evolving body of knowledge and research applications from nursing, social, physiological, and the basic sciences.

- Advances in nursing practice, health care delivery, and technology.

- Participation of nurses in intra- and interdisciplinary efforts that affect health care delivery systems.

- The numbers and variety of health personnel, health care consumer populations, and types of services provided in any given setting.

- Health care consumer, organizational, legislative, policy, regulatory, or professional development requirements.

- Increased focus on evidence-based practice outcomes.

- Political, social, economic, legislative, and regulatory factors that influence nursing and health care throughout the world.

Continuing Competence

Continuing competence is a hallmark of professionalism and a means by which a profession is held accountable to society. It is defined as "ongoing professional nursing competence according to level of expertise, responsibility, and domains of practice as evidenced by behavior based on beliefs, attitudes and knowledge matched to and in the context of a set of expected outcomes as defined by nursing scope of practice, policy, *Code of Ethics*, standards, guidelines, and benchmarks that assure safe performance of professional activities" (ANA January 2000, p. 16). A commitment to continuing competence mandates lifelong learning activities for all professional nurses.

Although the professional nurse remains ultimately responsible, the professional association, employers, credentialing bodies, providers of educational offerings, and regulatory agencies also share the responsibility for ensuring continuing competence. Professional nurses engage in appropriate professional development opportunities and activities to meet their immediate learning needs as well as those for future career goals. Employers, professional organizations, regulatory groups, and academic institutions can provide the means to assist with the accomplishment of this task. Discussion of the various responsibilities related to continuing competence were outlined in the Special 1999 ANA House of Delegates Background Report on Continued Competence (ANA June 1999b). See Appendix B for the chronology of ANA's continuing competence initiatives and Appendix C for responsibilities for continuing competence.

Framework for Nursing Professional Development

Nursing professional development is the lifelong process of active participation by nurses in learning activities that assist in developing and maintaining their continuing competence, enhance their professional practice, and support achievement of their career goals. Nursing professional development builds on the educational and experiential bases of nurses across their professional careers for the ultimate goal of ensuring the quality of health care to the public.

Nursing professional development activities can be described as existing in the domains of continuing education, staff development, and academic education. As shown in Figure 1, these areas overlap as individuals select the most effective way to meet their professional development needs and as educators engage in their practice roles. Staff development includes continuing education activities, academic education, or both as preparation for a particular role. Academic education may be accessed to pursue a specific course of study for a degree or certificate or as individual courses through which to update oneself in a particular area. Continuing education can be part of staff development, part of a formal academic program, or study in an accredited program for the purpose of enhancing nursing practice. The concepts of continuing competence and lifelong learning are central to all nursing professional development activities.

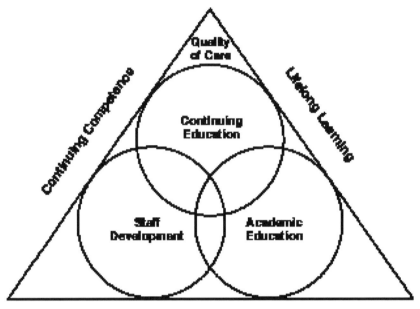

Figure 1. Framework for Nursing Professional Development

Continuing education refers to systematic professional learning experiences designed to augment the knowledge, skills, and attitudes of nurses and therefore enrich the nurses' contributions to quality health care and their pursuit of professional career goals. Some continuing education activities involve participant attendance where the pace of the activity is determined by the provider, who plans and schedules the activity. Other activities are designed for completion by the learner, independently, at the learner's own pace and at a time of the learner's choice.

Staff development is the systematic process of assessment, planning development, and evaluation that enhances the performance or professional development of health care providers and their continuing competence (National Nursing Staff Development Organization 1999). Staff development activities, which generally are sponsored by nurses' employers and focus on competence assessment and development, include continuing education, orientation, and in-service educational activities. New nursing staff members' competence is assessed, validated, and developed in orientation. Orientation socializes new nursing staff members, introducing them to the organizational culture and philosophy, goals, policies, role expectations, and other factors necessary to function in a specific work setting. In-service educational activities are those learning experiences designed to help nurses acquire, maintain, or increase their competence in fulfilling their responsibilities to deliver quality health care. As roles and responsibilities change, the need for continuing competence intensifies.

Academic education, as referred to in this framework, consists of courses taken for undergraduate or graduate credit in an institution of higher learning that may or may not lead to a degree or completion of a certificate program. Although professional development begins on entry into the basic nursing education program, for the purposes of this definition, academic education refers to those courses taken in colleges or universities after the basic nursing education program.

The nursing professional development educators may have expanded responsibilities for professional development that encompass ensuring continuing competence of other health care personnel within the agency, organization, or community.

SCOPE OF PRACTICE FOR NURSING PROFESSIONAL DEVELOPMENT

The scope of practice of nursing professional development has expanded along with the scope of nursing practice. Perhaps at no time in nursing's history has there been a greater need for competent, committed, and creative educators prepared for facilitating the achievement of learning needs by diverse learners. Furthermore, public concerns about the cost and quality of health care, consumer needs, and expectations of nurses add to the scope of practice and responsibilities of nursing professional development educators.

Nursing professional development is achieved in a wide variety of settings using numerous methodologies. Based on needs and values, learners determine the type and extent of the learning activities. Educational activities are directly influenced by an organization's missions, goals, values, priorities, and resources. In a competitive health care environment, educators must be proactive, take risks, and employ creativity. These factors, in turn, determine the dimension and scope of specific educational planning by individuals and employers.

Roles of Nursing Professional Development Educators

The roles of nursing professional development educators emerge from the standards of practice of professional development and have been conceptualized as those of educator, facilitator, change agent, consultant, researcher, and leader. In an environment of enhanced telecommunication resources and growing internationalism, nurse educators must appreciate the diversity in roles and functions of the international organizations, educational facilities, and agencies that directly or indirectly affect nursing professional development. Similarly, nurse educators must also be knowledgeable about the international differences in definitions of terms and requirements for continuing professional nursing competence, relicensure, certification, and recertification.

Educator Role

In the educator role, nursing professional development educators provide an appropriate climate for learning and facilitate the adult learning process. Educators ensure that learners are actively involved in the process of assessment of learning needs and outcomes and that educational standards are maintained. Educational activities, based on identified learner and organizational needs, are planned and presented by qualified faculty. Educators evaluate the effectiveness and outcomes of their educational endeavors and continually strive to plan activities that meet learner needs.

Educators and others collaborate with learners to enable them to develop portfolios that document the professional development of career planning and demonstrate learning and continuing competence. Portfolios, which include professional credentials, continuing education, leadership activities, and a narrative self-reflection of practice, document the relevance of nurses' professional learning experiences. Educators, along with others, assist the learners in documenting the key linkages of the elements of the portfolios to their continuing competence in practice and quality of care.

Regardless of the setting, educators develop, plan, and present educational activities within their areas of expertise and directly or indirectly foster the development of competence in the learner. Appropriate audiovisual aids, interactive teaching strategies, quality improvement techniques, and other resources are used to engage learners in critical thinking and problem solving. Educators also need a strong knowledge base of teaching and learning theories, curriculum design, test and measurement evaluation, research, and technological options to assist learners in achieving their goals and evaluating the outcomes of their professional developmental activities.

Facilitator Role

In the facilitator role, nursing professional development educators assist learners in identifying both their learning needs and the effective learning activities required to meet those needs. Facilitation may include providing time for individuals to meet their educational needs or guiding them to the appropriate resources. Nursing professional development educators frequently work with intra- or interdisciplinary teams, brainstorm and problem solve, and participate in strategic planning. Educators serve as role models for education and facilitate team building. They have a responsibility to foster a positive attitude about the benefits and opportunities of lifelong learning.

Change Agent Role

All nursing professional development educators serve as change agents at the organizational, community, state, national, or international levels. Nurses in all settings are being forced to cope with many changes, and the educator can help facilitate the initiation of, adoption of, and adaptation to change. Through leadership and participation in various activities such as committees, task forces, projects, and organizational strategic planning meetings, educators identify what changes should be made and can influence the necessary policy, procedures, or legislation to create the change.

Consultant Role

All educators act in a formal or informal consultant role. Such a role may involve assisting with the integration of new learning into the practice or educational environment. This role may include serving as a resource assisting nurses to design needed educational experiences. Consultative activities are provided to groups, departments, organizations, and other social entities by providing access to expertise. The consultant role includes assisting individuals and groups in defining problems, identifying available internal and external educational resources, and selecting educational options. In the consultant role, the educator provides feedback to the learners and the organization related to the effectiveness of the learning and the learning activity.

Researcher Role

Research is designed, created, and applied by the educator. The researcher role most often is implemented by integrating relevant research outcomes into nursing professional development practice through effective learning activities. Nursing professional development educators support the integration of research into practice and help develop staff members' knowledge and skills in the research process, as well as foster the use of systematic evaluative research with regard to clinical, educational, and managerial data. Nursing professional development educators also evaluate outcomes of educational endeavors and track learner outcomes as the profession moves to evidenced-based practice. The educators may also be active in the research process as principal investigators, collaborators, or evaluators.

Leader Role

The educator leadership role relates to providing and supporting organizational and administrative structures to achieve departmental and organizational goals. This role may include managing overall program activities, including human and monetary resources, and implementing effective negotiation skills. Educators ensure that educational activities are congruent with the organization's mission, vision, and goals and include an evaluation of the effectiveness of the overall educational programming. Communicating efficiently and effectively with all levels of the organization and using problem-solving skills are other aspects of the leadership role.

Educators also model behaviors that reflect participation and leadership in activities external to the organization, such as involvement in the professional association, specialty organizations, and the surrounding local, state, national, or international communities. Leaders demonstrate leadership by maintaining educational or clinical competencies appropriate to their role, reflecting their own professional growth and development. Educators integrate ethical principles in all aspects of practice.

Educational Preparation of Nursing Professional Development Educators

A professional development educator should have a graduate degree in nursing or a related specialty. If the graduate degree is in a related discipline, then the baccalaureate degree must be in nursing. Educators should demonstrate knowledge of relevant educational content and appropriate methods of delivery and the ability to develop and facilitate relevant and effective education for adult learners. Through self-evaluation and ongoing professional development, nurse educators develop, maintain, and enhance their expertise in testing and outcome measurement and evaluation, learning theories and principles, methodologies of delivery, knowledge of teaching, and other areas.

Because of the complexity of nursing and the health care environment, administrators of professional development departments should optimally have a doctoral degree in nursing or a related field, such as education. Minimally, the administrator of the department should have a master's degree. One of these degrees (baccalaureate, master's, or doctorate) must be in nursing. Administrators should demonstrate managerial, business, and educational knowledge and skills. The educational and management expertise of the administrator is developed, maintained, and enhanced through self-evaluation and ongoing professional development.

Lifelong learning is important for nursing professional development educators as a means for maintaining and increasing their competence and for their personal and professional growth. Certification for professional development educators and administrators is obtained by passing the certification examination in nursing professional development and includes a recertification option.

STANDARDS OF PRACTICE FOR NURSING PROFESSIONAL DEVELOPMENT

Standard I. Assessment

The nursing professional development educator collects pertinent information related to potential educational needs of the nurse.

Measurement Criteria

1. Data are collected from a variety of sources including, but not limited to, the nurse, professional organizations, consumers, nursing experts, reports on trends in the health care system, legislation, information about societal and organizational trends, and reports of advances in treatments and technology.

2. The educator establishes the data collection activities.

3. Pertinent data are collected using a variety of appropriate assessment techniques and instruments including, but not limited to, focus groups, questionnaires, evaluations of past programs, and analysis of trends.

4. Relevant data are documented in a retrievable form.

5. The data collection process is systematic and ongoing.

Standard II. Diagnosis: Analysis to Determine Target Audience and Learner Needs

The nursing professional development educator analyzes the assessment data to determine the target audience and the learner needs.

Measurement Criteria

1. The target audience and learner needs are derived from the assessment data.

2. Identified needs are validated with the nurse, consumer, content experts, and other educators when possible and appropriate.

3. Identified needs are documented in a manner that facilitates the determination of purpose statements, educational objectives, program content, and evaluation criteria.

Standard III. Identification of Educational Outcomes

The nursing professional development educator identifies the general purpose and educational objectives for each learning activity.

Measurement Criteria

1. General purpose statements and educational objectives are determined from the learner's identified needs and incorporate the principles of adult learning.

2. Educational objectives are mutually formulated among the nursing professional development educator, content expert(s), and the intended learners.

3. Educational objectives are culturally appropriate.

4. Educational objectives are realistic in relation to the learners' present and potential capabilities.

5. Educational objectives are attainable in relation to learning resources.

6. Educational objectives include a time estimate and explanation of the requirements for fulfillment.

7. Attainment of educational objectives will benefit the learners and consumers of nursing care.

8. Educational objectives are stated in behavioral terms and are written as measurable goals.

Standard IV. Planning

The nursing professional development educator identifies and collaborates with content experts to develop activities to facilitate learners' achievement of the educational objectives.

Measurement Criteria

1. The learning activity content is individualized to the target audience (e.g., basic education, experience, and preferred method of learning), the resources available, and the domains of learning.

2. The content is developed with input from the target audience.

3. The content reflects the educational objectives, as well as current and future nursing practice.

4. Adult learning and instructional design principles are reflected in planning.

5. The outline of the content is documented.

6. Interdisciplinary collaboration is encouraged and documented.

7. Budget planning for the program reflects sound business practices.

8. Marketing and promotional materials accurately reflect all aspects of the educational activity.

Standard V. Implementation

The nursing professional development educator ensures that the planned educational activities are implemented.

Measurement Criteria

1. The educational activity is consistent with the planned general purpose, educational objectives, and content outline.

2. The educational activity is implemented in a timely and appropriate manner.

3. Criteria for successful completion of the educational activity are provided to the learner and are documented.

4. Verification of completion of the educational activity is documented and available to the learner.

5. The educational activities are varied, interactive, and designed to meet the needs of the adult learner.

Standard VI. Evaluation

The nursing professional development educator conducts a comprehensive evaluation of the educational activity.

Measurement Criteria

1. Evaluation is systematic, ongoing, and criterion-based.

2. The educator, content experts, faculty, and learners are involved in the evaluation process, as appropriate.

3. Ongoing evaluation data are used to revise the purpose statement, educational objectives, content, method of delivery, and location of the educational activity, as needed.

4. Revisions to the purpose statement, educational objectives, content, method of delivery, and location of the educational activity are documented.

5. The effectiveness of the learning activity is evaluated in relation to the learner's achievement of the educational objectives and the development of the individual nurse's portfolio, which includes documentation of ongoing professional development, career planning, and continuing professional nursing development.

6. A summary of the evaluation responses and achievement of outcomes is documented and shared with the appropriate persons, such as content experts, presenters, and the planning committee.

7. Future planning of educational activities incorporates evaluation data.

STANDARDS OF PROFESSIONAL PERFORMANCE FOR NURSING PROFESSIONAL DEVELOPMENT

Standard I. Quality of Nursing Professional Development Practice

The nursing professional development educator systematically evaluates the quality and effectiveness of nursing professional development practice.

Measurement Criteria

The nursing professional development educator

1. Identifies aspects of nursing professional development practice important for quality monitoring.

2. Identifies indicators used to monitor quality and effectiveness of nursing professional development practice.

3. Collects data to monitor quality and effectiveness of nursing professional development practice.

4. Analyzes quality data to identify opportunities for improving nursing professional development practice.

5. Evaluates learning activities.

6. Formulates recommendations to improve nursing professional development practice or outcomes.

7. Implements activities to enhance the quality of nursing professional development practice.

8. Participates on intra- and interdisciplinary teams that evaluate professional development.

9. Develops, implements, and evaluates policies and procedures to improve the quality of nursing professional development practice.

Standard II. Performance Appraisal

The nursing professional development educator evaluates his or her own nursing practice in relation to professional practice standards, relevant statutes and regulations, and maintenance of continuing professional nursing competence.

Measurement Criteria

1. The nursing professional development educator

    a. Engages in a performance appraisal on a regular basis, identifying areas of strength as well as areas in which further professional development would be beneficial.

    b. Seeks constructive feedback regarding his or her own practice.

    c. Takes action to achieve goals identified during the performance appraisal.

    d. Participates in peer review as appropriate.

2. The educator's practice reflects knowledge of current professional practice standards, laws, and regulations.

Standard III. Education

The nursing professional development educator acquires and maintains current knowledge and competency in nursing professional development practice.

Measurement Criteria

The nursing professional development educator

1. Participates in ongoing educational activities related to practice knowledge and professional issues.

2. Acquires knowledge and skills appropriate to the specialty area, practice setting, and cultural competence.

3. Seeks experiences that reflect current theories and methods of teaching, learning, and delivery.

4. Maintains a personal portfolio that documents ongoing continuing professional nursing competence.

5. Seeks certification when eligible.

Standard IV. Collegiality

The nursing professional development educator interacts with, and contributes to the professional development of, peers and other health care providers as colleagues.

Measurement Criteria

The nursing professional development educator

1.   Shares knowledge and skills with colleagues.

2.   Provides peers with constructive feedback regarding their practice.

3.   Interacts with colleagues to enhance his or her own professional nursing practice.

4.   Contributes to an environment that is conducive to the education of students, peers, colleagues, and others.

5.   Serves as a model in the roles of educator, facilitator, change agent, consultant, researcher, and leader to promote the professional growth of peers.

6.   Contributes to a supportive and healthy work environment that fosters mutual respect.

Standard V. Ethics

The nursing professional development educator's decisions and actions are based on ethical principles.

Measurement Criteria

The nursing professional development educator

1.   Integrates ethical principles into the practice of nursing professional development.

2.   Uses the American Nurses Association's *Code for Nurses with Interpretive Statements* (ANA 1985), *Scope and Standards of Practice for Nursing Professional Development,* and other appropriate standards, guidelines, and benchmarks to guide practice.

3. Maintains confidentiality within legal and regulatory parameters.

4. Safeguards learners' rights related to the educational process.

5. Is sensitive to the boundaries of individual or organizational ownership of educational and program materials developed as part of the educator's fulfillment of work responsibilities.

6. Properly credits colleagues' work, both published and unpublished.

7. Gives assurance that promotional materials accurately represent the educational activity.

8. Obtains permission from the owner before duplicating an educational activity.

9. Practices in a manner that is sensitive to cultural diversity.

10. Engages in activities that do not constitute a conflict of interest.

11. Follows appropriate guidelines for commercial support of educational programs.

12. Can accurately identify an ethical dilemma and seek appropriate ethical consultation as necessary.

13. Is cognizant of the topics and content in the fields of bioethics and nursing ethics.

Standard VI. Collaboration

The nursing professional development educator collaborates with others in the practice of nursing professional development at the institutional, local, regional, state, national, or international levels.

Measurement Criteria

The nursing professional development educator

1. Collaborates with organizations and other professionals in teaching, consultation, management, research, leadership, facilitation, and change agent activities.

2. Collaborates with agencies and organizations as needed to achieve mutual educational goals.

3. Makes referrals, including provisions for continuity of education.

Standard VII. Research

The nursing professional development educator participates in and uses evidence-based research to identify strategies for improving professional development activities, nursing practice, and patient outcomes.

Measurement Criteria

The nursing professional development educator

1. Uses available evidence, including research data, in the educational process.

2. Participates in research activities as appropriate. Such activities may include

   • Identifying problems suitable for nursing professional development research.

   • Serving as principal investigator, collaborator, or evaluator.

   • Participating in data collection.

   • Participating in a unit, organization, or community research committee or program.

   • Conducting research.

   • Sharing research activities with others.

   • Critiquing research for application to practice.

   • Using research findings in the development of policies, procedures, and guidelines.

Standard VIII. Management and Resource Utilization

The nursing professional development educator considers factors related to safety, effectiveness, and cost in planning, delivering, and managing nursing professional development activities.

Measurement Criteria

The nursing professional development educator

1. Develops a financial plan sufficient to meet educational needs.

2. Advocates and plans for available and appropriate support services for educational activities.

3. Effectively administers the human resources, facilities, materials, equipment, and technologies used for educational purposes.

4. Provides for the evaluation of the appropriateness and effectiveness of material resources and facilities as a component of each educational activity.

5. Provides an appropriate climate for learning that facilitates the adult learning process and maintenance of continuing professional nursing competence.

6. Ensures that educational programs are congruent with organizational goals and are based on identified needs.

7. Evaluates factors related to safety, effectiveness, availability, and cost when choosing education options.

8. Maintains a record-keeping and report system that

   - Documents all aspects of educational activities in compliance with departmental, organizational, and external agency requirements.

   - Establishes mechanisms for systematic, easy retrieval of data on educational activities and participants.

   - Maintains confidentiality of records.

   - Provides periodic reports to appropriate organizational and agency representatives to document and evaluate progress toward attainment of organizational goals.

Standard IX. Leadership

The nursing professional development educator practices in a manner that provides leadership in the work setting as well as the profession.

Measurement Criteria

The nursing professional development educator

1. Serves in key roles in the work setting by serving on committees, councils, and administrative teams.

2. Monitors educational, clinical practice, legislative and regulatory, organizational, and health care delivery systems, issues, and trends.

3. Incorporates new models, techniques, and theories related to nursing professional development and clinical practice.

4. Provides guidance, resources, and knowledge for professional growth of others.

5. Participates in professional nursing organizations and the community.

GLOSSARY

Academic education—Courses taken for undergraduate or graduate credit in an institution of higher learning that may or may not lead to a degree or completion of a certificate program. Although professional development begins on entry into the basic nursing education program, for the purposes of this definition, academic education refers to those courses taken in colleges or universities after the basic nursing education program.

Adult learning principles—The basis for or the beliefs underlying the teaching and learning approaches to adults as learners based on recognition of the adult individual's autonomy and self-direction, life experiences, readiness to learn, and problem orientation to learning. Approaches include mutual, respectful collaboration of educators and learners in the assessment, planning, implementation, and evaluation of educational activities.

Certification—The process by which a professional organization validates, based on predetermined standards, an individual registered nurse's qualifications, knowledge, and practice in a defined functional or clinical area of nursing.

Content—Subject matter of educational activity that relates to the educational objectives.

Content expert—An individual with documented qualifications that demonstrate education, knowledge, and experience in a particular subject matter.

Continuing competence—Ongoing professional nursing competence according to level of expertise, responsibility, and domains of practice as evidenced by behavior based on beliefs, attitudes, and knowledge matched to and in the context of a set of expected outcomes as defined by nursing scope of practice, policy, code of ethics, standards, guidelines, and benchmarks that ensure safe performance of professional activities.

Continuing education—Systematic professional learning experiences designed to augment the knowledge, skills, and attitudes of nurses and therefore enrich the nurses' contributions to quality health care and their pursuit of professional career goals.

Distance learning—A formal educational activity in which most of the instruction occurs when the learner and the educator are not in the same place. The instruction may take place either synchronously (at the same time) (e.g., interactive video) or asynchronously (at different times) (e.g., online/Internet or correspondence courses).

Domains of learning—Three areas in which learning takes place: the cognitive, psychomotor, and affective.

Educational activity—A planned, organized effort aimed at accomplishing educational objectives.

Educational objectives—A statement of the learner outcome(s) of an educational activity that is measurable and achievable within the designated time frame.

Evaluation—The process of determining significance or quality by systematic appraisal and study.

Evaluation criteria—Relevant, measurable indicators of significant or quality standards.

In-service educational activities—Learning experiences provided in the work setting for the purpose of assisting staff members in performing their assigned functions in that particular agency or institution.

Needs—Discrepancy between what is desired and what exists.

Nursing professional development—The lifelong process of active participation by nurses in learning activities that assist in developing and maintaining their continuing competence, enhance their professional practice, and support achievement of their career goals.

Nursing professional development educator—A registered nurse whose practice is in nursing education and who facilitates lifelong learning in a variety of health care, educational, and academic settings.

Orientation—The process of introducing nursing staff to the philosophy, goals, policies, procedures, role expectations, and other factors needed to function in a specific work setting. Orientation takes place both for new employees and when changes in nurses' roles, responsibilities, and practice settings occur.

Outcome—The end result of a learning activity measured by written evaluation or change in practice.

Patient—Recipient of nursing care. The term patient rather than client is used in this document and may represent an individual, family or group, or community.

Portfolio—Material documenting the professional development, career planning, demonstration of learning, and maintenance of continuing professional nursing competence of the individual nurse.

Purpose statement—A statement describing why and for whom an educational activity has been designed.

Self-directed learning—An approach to learning in which the learner takes the initiative and responsibility for identifying learning needs and sets the pace for the learning process. The learning activity or process may be designed by the learner or others and may or may not be planned or structured. Self-directed learning methods might include, but are not limited to, computer-assisted instruction, Internet courses, and self-learning packages.

Staff development—The systematic process of assessment, development, and evaluation that enhances the performance or professional development of health care providers and their continuing competence (National Nursing Staff Development Organization 1999).

Standards of nursing practice—Authoritative statements that describe a level of care or performance common to the profession of nursing by which the quality of nursing practice can be judged and reassured.

Standards of professional performance—Authoritative statements that describe a competent level of behavior in the professional role, including activities related to quality of care, performance appraisal, education, collegiality, ethics, collaboration, research, and resource utilization.

Target audience—Group for which an educational activity has been designed.

APPENDIX A

Chronology of the Evolution of Nursing Professional Development

1969   First national conference on nursing continuing education held in Williamsburg, Virginia, to provide a forum for discussion of national issues by college and university providers of nursing continuing education (Cooper 1980, DeSilets 1998).

1972   Commission on Continuing Education is established by American Nurses Association (ANA) (ANA 1972b).

1973   Article about Continuing Education Council membership published (Continuing Education Council Seeks Members 1973).

1974   *Standards for Continuing Education in Nursing* published (ANA 1974).

1975   *Accreditation of Continuing Education in Nursing* published (ANA 1975).

First members of the National Accreditation Board, the National Review Committee, and five regional accrediting committees appointed by ANA's Commission on Nursing Education (ANA Accreditation Board Appointed 1975).

1976   *Continuing Education in Nursing: An Overview* published (ANA 1976a).

Guidelines for Staff Development published (ANA 1976b).

1978   *Self-Directed Continuing Education in Nursing* published (ANA 1978b).

Guidelines for Staff Development revised (ANA 1978a); national workshops held to facilitate implementation in practice, which provided first recognition of evolving field of staff development in practice settings and its complement to nursing continuing education in academic settings.

1979   *Continuing Education in Nursing: An Overview* published (ANA 1979).

1984   *Standards for Continuing Education in Nursing* published (ANA 1984).

1989   Name for ANA Council on Continuing Education changed to Council on Continuing Education and Staff Development to more clearly reflect expansion of the field of specialty practice in nursing education (ANA April 1989).

National Nursing Staff Development Organization (NNSDO) established and incorporated.

1990   *Standards for Nursing Staff Development* published (ANA 1990).

1991   American Nurses Credentialing Center (ANCC) established as a subsidiary of ANA to implement the credentialing programs (including certification for nurses and accreditation of continuing education) (ANCC 1996).

1992   Certification in nursing continuing education and staff development first offered by ANCC in collaboration with NNSDO (ANA 1992b).

Roles and Responsibilities for Nursing Continuing Education and Staff Development Across All Settings published (ANA 1992a).

1994   *Standards for Nursing Professional Development: Continuing Education and Staff Development* published (ANA 1994).

1995   Name of the ANA Council changed to Council for Nursing Professional Education and Development.

1997   *Report of the ANA Council/NNSDO Task Force on Advanced Practice in Nursing Continuing Education and Staff Development* (1997) published.

1999   ANA Council for Nursing Professional Education and Development dissolved by action of ANA House of Delegates as part of revision to overall organizational structure (ANA 1999a, ANA Creates New "House" for all Nurses 1999).

APPENDIX B

Chronology of American Nurses Association's Continuing Competence Initiatives

1972   House of Delegates issued two position/policy statements: "A Continued Clinical Competence of Faculty in Schools of Nursing" (1972a) and "Preparation for Primary Health Care Practitioners" (1972c).

1978, 1980   House of Delegates established a mechanism for the development of the roles, functions, and competencies of the two categories of nursing practice.

1978   American Nurses Association (ANA) Council of State Boards of Nursing abolished June 5.

National Council of State Boards of Nursing convened first meeting June 6.

1985   ANA published *Code for Nurses with Interpretive Statements* (ANA 1985).

1996   House of Delegates issued policy/position statement: "Regulation and Licensure of Professional Nurses in the Health Care Work Force" (ANA 1996).

1997   American Academy of Nursing (AAN) convened the "Nursing Futures and Regulation Conference."

1998   ANA House of Delegates issued "Status Report on Competence" (ANA 1998a).

ANCC began a five-year longitudinal study to determine whether the credentialing process could be used to measure continued competency for two categories of nurse practitioners (adult and family) for purposes of certification.

June 1999 ANA conducted the Continuing Education Issues Forum on Continued Competency at the House of Delegates meeting with invited experts presenting (ANA June 1999b).

Fall 1999 ANA appointed an expert panel of representatives from the state nurses associations, National Council of State Boards of Nursing, American Nurses Foundation, AAN, ANCC, and others to develop the Policy of Continued Competency, research recommendations, and the progressive plan of action.

Winter 2000 ANA Expert Panel on Continuing Competence

- Reviewed reports and recommendations from regulatory and private entities at the national and international levels, other professional associations, and accrediting bodies calling for the development and implementation of a continuing competence program.

- Identified assumptions and definitions of "continuing competence" and "continuing professional nursing competence (CPNC)."

- Developed the elements of the CPNC process and portfolio to include professional credentials, organization and workplace continuing education, leadership, and narrative self-reflection.

- Reviewed legal considerations.

- Created guidelines of CPNC process and portfolio.

- Designed the research agenda, the research questions, and the pilot program to test and refine the model of the CPNC process and portfolio.

- Identified long-range plans for seeking funding and collaborating with other key stakeholders within and external to the profession to assist in the implementation of the model.

March 2000 The draft report and recommendations of ANA's Expert Panel on Continuing Competence were provided to the ANA Board of Directors.

APPENDIX C

Responsibilities for Continuing Competence

Responsibilities of the Individual Nurse

Each nurse has the personal responsibility to maintain competency in practice by maintaining currency of knowledge and skills (ANA 1985). Nurses are accountable for identifying their learning needs. They are ultimately responsible for seeking appropriate educational experiences and for ensuring that they comply with the rules and regulations of the current nurse practice act within the state in which they are practicing.

Nurses must also be willing to have their practice reviewed and evaluated by their peers. The nurses' professional profiles or portfolios can enhance these evaluations and reviews. Validation of successful completion of nursing professional development program activities constitutes an important part of this evidence. In addition, individuals may become certified by a recognized accrediting body as another mechanism to demonstrate their continuing competence.

Responsibilities of the Professional Association

The continuing competence of nurses is critical to safe, quality health care. ANA and its constituencies, as the professional association, assist registered nurses in remaining competent by developing professional practice standards. The performance and competency of registered nurses are based and measured on these professional practice standards. ANA also provides continuing education programs, influences changes in nurse practice acts, and cooperates with certification agencies. Furthermore, ANA monitors the systems that affect the practice of nursing, influences legislation and health policy through its legislative program, and supports nursing research that links nursing professional development to nursing interventions and patient outcomes. Increasingly, these activities incorporate dialogue about nursing professional development activities among international educational facilities, agencies, and organizations, such as the International Council of Nurses.

Responsibilities of the Employer

The work setting and staffing patterns influence the ability of registered nurses to competently deliver care. Employers have obligations to provide an environment for the provision of safe quality care. They must meet the requirements of accrediting bodies to ensure the ongoing competencies of employees. When introducing new technologies, systems, policies, and procedures, employers provide educational opportunities for staff to ensure the best practice and, ultimately, the highest quality of care. Employers validate the credentials with regard to academic preparation, licensure, and certification(s).

Responsibilities of Regulatory Agencies

State boards of nursing are required to protect the health and safety of the public through the initiation and maintenance of licensure held by professional nurses. Boards of nursing interpret, administer, and enforce nurse practice acts and rules and regulations. Regulatory bodies and agencies establish guidelines to ensure workers are competent and perform in a safe manner, avoiding injury to themselves and their patients or clients.

REFERENCES

American Nurses Association (ANA). 1965. *Standards for Organized Nursing Services in Hospitals, Public Health Agencies, Nursing Homes, Industries, and Clinics.* New York: American Nurses Association.

American Nurses Association (ANA). 1972a. A Continued Clinical Competence of Faculty in Schools of Nursing. In House of Delegates Report. Kansas City, Mo.: American Nurses Association.

American Nurses Association (ANA). 1972b. House of Delegates Reports 1970–1972. Kansas City, Mo.: American Nurses Association.

American Nurses Association (ANA). 1972c. Preparation for Primary Health Care Practitioners. In House of Delegates Report. Kansas City, Mo.: American Nurses Association.

American Nurses Association (ANA). 1973. *Standards of Nursing Practice.* Kansas City, Mo.: American Nurses Association.

American Nurses Association (ANA). 1974. *Standards for Continuing Education in Nursing.* Kansas City, Mo.: American Nurses Association.

American Nurses Association (ANA). 1975. *Accreditation of Continuing Education in Nursing.* Kansas City, Mo.: American Nurses Association.

American Nurses Association (ANA). 1976a. *Continuing Education in Nursing: An Overview.* Kansas City, Mo.: American Nurses Association.

American Nurses Association (ANA). 1976b. *Guidelines for Staff Development.* Kansas City, Mo.: American Nurses Association.

American Nurses Association (ANA). 1978a. *Guidelines for Staff Development.* Rev. Kansas City, Mo.: American Nurses Association.

American Nurses Association (ANA). 1978b. *Self-Directed Continuing Education in Nursing.* Kansas City, Mo.: American Nurses Association.

American Nurses Association (ANA). 1979. *Continuing Education in Nursing: An Overview.* Kansas City, Mo.: American Nurses Association.

American Nurses Association (ANA). 1984. *Standards for Continuing Education in Nursing.* Kansas City, Mo.: American Nurses Association.

American Nurses Association (ANA). 1985. *Code for Nurses with Interpretive Statements.* Kansas City, Mo.: American Nurses Association.

American Nurses Association (ANA). April 1989. Board of Directors Minutes. Kansas City, Mo.: American Nurses Association.

American Nurses Association (ANA). 1990. *Standards for Nursing Staff Development.* Kansas City, Mo.: American Nurses Association.

American Nurses Association (ANA). 1992a. *Roles and Responsibilities for Nursing Continuing Education and Staff Development Across All Settings.* Washington, D.C.: American Nurses Association.

American Nurses Association (ANA). 1992b. House of Delegates Summary of Proceedings. Washington, D.C.: American Nurses Association.

American Nurses Association (ANA). 1994. *Standards for Nursing Professional Development: Continuing Education and Staff Development.* Washington, D.C.: American Nurses Association.

American Nurses Association (ANA). 1995. *Nursing's Social Policy Statement.* Washington, D.C.: American Nurses Association.

American Nurses Association (ANA). 1996. Regulation and Licensure of Professional Nurses in the Health Care Work Force. Washington, D.C.: American Nurses Association, House of Delegates.

American Nurses Association (ANA). 1998a. Status Report on Competence. Washington, D.C.: American Nurses Association, House of Delegates.

American Nurses Association (ANA). 1998b. *Standards of Clinical Nursing Practice.* 2d ed. Washington, D.C.: American Nurses Association.

American Nurses Association (ANA). 1999a. House of Delegates Report. Washington, D.C.: American Nurses Association.

American Nurses Association (ANA). June 1999b. Special 1999 House of Delegates Background Report on Continued Competence (Policy Series No. 98-BAC-05). Washington, D.C.: American Nurses Association.

American Nurses Association (ANA). January 2000. Continuing Competence: Nursing's Agenda for the 21st Century (draft). Washington, D.C.: American Nurses Association, Expert Panel on Continuing Competence.

American Nurses Credentialing Center (ANCC). 1996. *American Nurses Credentialing Center's Commission on Accreditation Manual for Accreditation as a Provider of Continuing Education in Nursing.* Washington, D.C.: American Nurses Association.

ANA Accreditation Board Appointed. 1975. *The American Nurse* 9(1):12.

ANA Creates New "House" for all Nurses. 1999. *The American Nurse* 4(31):1,8.

Continuing Education Council Seeks Members. 1973. *The American Nurse,* 1(1):1.

Cooper, S. S. 1980. The Past as Prologue. In *Perspectives in Continuing Education.* Edited by S. S. Cooper and M. C. Neal. Pacific Palisades, Ca.: NURSECO.

DeSilets, L. D. 1998. Accreditation of Continuing Education: The Critical Elements. *The Journal of Continuing Education in Nursing* 29(5):204–210.

National Nursing Staff Development Organization. 1999. *Strategic Plan 2000.* Pensacola, Fl.: National Nursing Staff Development Organization.

Report of the ANA Council/NNSDO Task Force on Advanced Practice in Nursing Continuing Education and Staff Development. 1997. Pensacola, Fl.: National Nursing Staff Development Organization.

INDEX

Page entries in this index from this book's 2000 edition, Scope and Standards of Practice for Nursing Professional Development, are marked by [2000].

A

academic liaison as NPD practice element, 16–17
academic partnerships, 7, 11, 21
  defined, 43
  See also partnerships in NPD
accountability in NPD practice, 10, 18, 19, 32, 39
advisor role in NPD practice, 18
advocacy, 18–19
  professional performance standard, 39
American Nurses Association (ANA), v, 18
  competence responsibilities and initiatives, [2000] 88–90
  [2000] 59, 87, 89
American Nurses Credentialing Center (ANCC), 21, 52
  [2000] 87, 88
assessment
  of professional competency, 3, 6, 19
  identification of trends and issues and, 22
  standard of practice, 23
  [2000] 71

C

career development, 6, 10
  evaluating competency, 13
  as NPD specialist responsibility, 10
certification, 8, 12, 13
change in educational process, 7
  influencing, 8, 30
  leading, 15, 17
  [2000] 68
clinical practice, changes in, 20–21
collaboration, 4, 11, 15–16
  in measurement criteria, 27, 30
  as NPD practice element, 17–18
  professional performance standard, 36
  [2000] 78–79

collegiality, professional performance standard, 35
  [2000] 77
competencies for NPD specialist, 13–15
competencies (core) in nursing, 12, 13–15
  defined, 43
competence and competencies, 1, 4
  assessment in NPD, 3, 6, 19
  core, 12, 13–15, 43
  defined, 43
  evaluating, standard for, 34
  measuring, 6
  in professional role, 8, 45
  programs, 5–6
  [2000] 61–63, 88–89, 76–77, 90–91
competency programs, 5–6
  defined, 43
compliance initiatives as NPD responsibility, 12
confidentiality in NPD practice, 14, 19
consultation, 11, 15
  role in NPD practice, 17–18
  standard of practice, 30
continuing education, 2, 12
  defined, 43
  types, 6
  [2000] 63–64, 87
coordination in NPD practice 5–7 *passim*
  standard of practice, 28
criteria for standards. *See* measurement criteria
cultural competence and diversity, 4, 14, 18–19, 34

D

data collection and usage in NPD practice, 8, 11, 19, 23, 27
delivery methods in NPD practice, 13, 16

diversity, 18, 19, 20, 37
  adapting education to, [2000] 61
  respecting, 19
documentation in NPD practice, 8, 11,
    16
  in measurement criteria, 23, 24, 26,
      27, 28, 32, 36, 38, 41
  portfolios as, [2000] 64, 67, 74, 76, 80

E
education and NPD practice
  academic, [2000] 63, [2000] 65
  continuing, 2, 6, 12, 43, [2000] 63–64,
      87
  coordination of, 28
evaluating competency, 14
  in-service, 6
  requirements for NPD specialty, 12
  responsibilities for NPD specialty,
      10–11
  standard of practice, 33
  [2000] 62, 63, 65, 67, 72–74, 76–77
  See also nurse educator
educator as NPD practice element,
    16–17
environments in NPD practice
  learning and practice, 9–10, 16–18,
      29
  NPD and learning, 4
ethics and ethical issues in NPD practice,
    14, 18, 19
  advocacy and, 18–19
  confidentialty in, 4, 9
  professional performance standard,
      37–38
  [2000] 77–78
evaluation in NPD practice, 31
  standard of practice, 34
  [2000] 74–76
evaluation of professional practice
  professional performance standard,
      34
evidence-based practice (EBP), 2, 3, 15,
    17, 18, 21, 23, 27
  defined, 43
  practice-based evidence and, 1, 5
  See also nursing research

F
facilitator role of NPD specialist, 1, 3–5,
    13–15 *passim*
  as NPD practice element, 16–17

G
generational issues in NPD practice,
    19, 20

H
health care, current and future NPD
    issues in, 19–21

I
identification of issues and trends
    professional performance standard,
      24
Identification of outcomes,
    professional performance standard, 25
implementation
  coordination and, 37
  nursing practice standard, 27
  [2000], 73
in-service education, 6
  definition, 43
interdisciplinary teams in health care,
    23, 42, 43
  defined, 43
interprofessional teams in health care,
    17, 35
  defined, 43–44
issues and trends in NPD, 19–21

K
knowledge base of NPD, 16
  maintaining, 33

L
laws, statutes, and regulations in NPD
    practice, 2, 4, 25
  compliance, 9, 12, 14
  ethics and, 37–38
  professional practice evaluation and,
      34
leadership, 12, 18
  educators, [2000] 69
  evaluating competency, 14–15

professional performance standard, 42
  as NPD specialist responsibility, 11
  transformational, 4, 46
learners, 4–5
  defined, 44
  respecting cultural diversity, 19
  [2000] 71–72
leaner-directed continuing education, 6
  defined, 44
leaner-paced continuing education, 6
  defined, 44
learning, 2, 7–8
  process, 15–16
  technology and, 15–16
learning environments in NPD, 2, 4
  defined, 44
  practice environments and, 9–10,
    16–18
  practice standard, 29
lifelong learning and NPD, 1, 3, 4, 13
  defined, 44
  [2000] 70

M

management (program and project),
    11, 15
measurement criteria
  standards of performance, 32–42,
    [2000] 75–81
  standards of practice, 23–31, [2000]
    71–74
mentors and mentoring in NPD practice,
    11, 13, 30, 32
  defined, 44
  as NPD practice element, 18
model of nursing professional
    development, 3

N

National Nursing Staff Development
    Organization (NNSDO), v, 52
nurse educators, 13, 16–17
  NPD specialist as,
  [2000] 61, 66–71
nursing education. *See* education
nursing professional development (NPD),
    1, 8

chronology of and literature, 51–52
determining target audience, 71–72
enhancing quality of, 32
evolution of practice, 2–3
learning environment , 2, 4, 9–10,
    16–18, 29
models, 3, 5
practice environments, 4, 9–10, 16–18,
    29
as practice specialty, 3
quality of practice, 32, [2000] 75
standards of performance, 32–42,
    [2000] 75–81
standards of practice, 23–31, [2000]
    71–74
[2000] 60–65
nursing professional development (NPD)
    specialists, 1–4
change agent role, 8, 15, 17, 30, [2000]
    68
core competencies for, 13–15
current role and evolution of, 9
defined, 44
education and qualifications of, 12–13
knowledge base, 16, 33
practice elements, 1, 15–18
practice model, 3f
role in adapting to healthcare
    evolution, 20
roles of, 1, 15
scope of responsibility, 10–12
self-evaluation and, 34, [2000] 75–76
standards of performance, 32–42
    [2000] 75–81
standards of practice, 23–42
    [2000] 60, 71–74
See also nurse educators
Nursing Professional Development
    Systems Model, 3
nursing research, 17–18
  integrating into practice, 40
  [2000] 68, 97
  See also research; researcher

O

orientation process, 5
  defined, 45

outcomes in NPD practice, 9, 10, 14, 16, 17, 25
  collaboration and, 36
  defined, 45
  evaluation and, 21
  measurement (defined), 45
  in NPD model, 3, 4, 7, 8
  planning and, 26
  practice standard (outcomes identification), 25
  resource utilization and, 41

P

partners in NPD (defined), 45
partnerships (academic),
partnerships in NPD, 34, 35, 36, 42
  academic partnerships, 11, 21, 43
  collegiality and, 35
peer review, 11, 34
  defined, 45
  [2000] 90
performance appraisal, [2000] 75–76
performance assessment in NPD, 4, 6, 18
performance standards. *See* standards of professional performance
performance
  role competence, 8
  assessing, 4, 6
plans and planning in NPD practice
  evaluation, 31
  implementation and, 27, 28, 29
  leadership and. 42
  standard of practice, 26
  succession, 46
  [2000] 72–73
portfolios as documentation in NPD, [2000] 64, 67, 74, 76, 80
  See also documentation
practice elements of NPD, 15–18
  examples, 16–18
practice environments in NPD, 4, 9–10
  defined, 44
  learning environments and, 9–10, 16–18
  practice standard, 29

practice-based evidence (PBE), 11
  defined, 45
  evidence-based practice and, 5
practice-to-science model, 5
professional competence. *See* competence and competencies
professional development. *See* nursing professional development; staff development
professional role competence, 8
  defined, 45
professional performance standard, 34
professional practice environments. *See* practice environments
program and project management
  evaluating competency in, 15
  as NPD responsibility . 11
provider-directed continuing education, 6
  defined, 45

Q

quality care and NPD, 2, 3, 6, 7, 9, 20
quality of NPD practice, 2, 10, 25
  professional performance standard, 32
  [2000] 75

R

regulatory issues *See* laws, statutes, regulations and in NPD practice
research and NPD practice, 5, 7
  professional performance standard, 40
  See also evidence-based practice; nursing research
researcher as NPD practice element, 17–18
resource utilization professional performance standard, 41
  [2000] 80
responsibility, scope of NPD , 10–12

S

scholarship in NPD practice, 7
science-to-service model, 5
Scope and Standards of Practice for Nursing Professional Development (2000), 59, 60,

scope of practice for NPD, 9–21
  advocacy, and ethics, 18–19
  educational preparation and
    qualifications, 12–14
  elements of practice, 15–18
  practice and learning environments,
    9–10
  scope of responsibility, 10–12
  trends and issues, 19–21
  [2000] 66–70
scope of responsibility of NPD specialist,
    10–12
self-assessment in NPD, 13
self-evaluation, 34
  [2000] 75–76
simulation in NPD practice, 10, 11, 21
  defined, 46
specialty certification, 8
staff development, v
  changes in, 2–3, 21
  as NPD domain, 2
  [2000] 63–64
staff issues in NPD future, 20
standards of practice, 23–31
  assessment, 23
  consultation, 30
  coordination, 28
  evaluation, 34
  implementation, 27
  issues and trends identification, 24
  learning and practice environment, 29
  outcomes identification, 25
  planning, 26

[2000], 71–74
  See also each standard
standards of professional performance,
    32–42
  advocacy, 39
  collaboration, 36
  collegiality, 35
  education, 33
  ethics, 37–38
  leadership, 42
  professional practice evaluation, 34
  quality of NPD practice, 32
  research, 40
  resource utilization, 41
  [2000], 75–81
  See also each standard.
students. *See* learners
succession planning, 6, 20
  defined, 46
systems model of nursing professional
    development, 3

T
team member as NPD practice element,
    17
technological issues in NPD practice, 1,
    2, 15, 16, 19
transformational nursing leadership, 4
  defined, 46
trends and issues in NPD practice, 19–21

W
workforce issues in NPD future, 20